The Brainstorms Healer
Epilepsy in Our Experience

*Stories of Health Care Professionals as
Care Providers and Patients*

COMMENTS ON
BRAINSTORMS:
EPILEPSY IN OUR WORDS

. . . the essence of the book . . . has fulfilled the author's intent to alleviate from those patients with seizures who have a sense of isolation the fear of feeling they are insane or crazy because of their weird experiences. It indicates that there are others having similar unusual experiences and they may even find a description of a seizure in there which is similar to their own.

Linda Moretti Ojeman
Electroencephalography and Clinical Neurophysiology

You cannot imagine how much it (the book) has helped me to accept epilepsy as something I'm just going to have to live with. Just knowing that I'm not the only one that has gone through some of these experiences makes it easier.

A Reader

This is an interesting and valuable little book in which Steven Schachter shares with us the experiences of his epilepsy patients in their own words. . . In no area of neurology is the history more important than in epilepsy, not only in making a correct diagnosis but in understanding the patient as a human being and partner in the therapeutic process.

Neurology

This is a wonderful book. Dr. Schachter has done a great service to epilepsy patients and their doctors, particularly the former, in compiling this comprehensive collection of the experiences of those suffering this unique disorder ... and in their own words. The seizure descriptions detail the rich fabric of human experience as reflected in the epileptic process . . . [they] attest to the often bizarre nature of epileptic symptoms, the pain inflicted, the loneliness of the experience, and the remarkable courage of these patients.

A. James Rowan, M.D.
Professor of Neurology
Mount Sinai School of Medicine
Chief, Neurology Service
Bronx DVA Medical Center

COMMENTS ON
THE BRAINSTORMS COMPANION:
EPILEPSY IN OUR VIEW

Books about epilepsy are not often emotional, nor do they usually elicit empathy. Indeed, they usually [only] cover the hard facts of the illness. This book is different. . . . These accounts of seizures remind us of the tremendous drama of witnessing them.

This is a very helpful book for patients, their relatives, and others who might witness seizures, as well as for the medical profession, especially those treating patients with epilepsy. It will enable us to deal better with the patient and the family and will no doubt increase our understanding into the emotional challenge of having epilepsy.

Elinor Ben-Menachem, Epilepsia

This book describes well the views and feelings of those who live with persons with epilepsy. It will enable physicians, care-givers, and educators . . . to better understand and to respond appropriately [to seizures]. . . . This is an excellent book of descriptions and views, and provides invaluable advice for physicians, care-givers, and paramedics.

Th. de Barsy, Extrait De La Revue Des Questions Scientifiques

I would recommend that all patients with epilepsy own a copy of this book. It should also be included in medical bookstores and medical and community libraries.

Tonya F. Fuller, Doody's Health Sciences Book Review Journal

COMMENTS ON
THE BRAINSTORMS FAMILY:
EPILEPSY ON OUR TERMS

Your book makes us epilepsy survivors feel part of a large family and not like we're struggling on our own.

A Reader

Families whose children are affected by epilepsy will find in this small but very appropriate volume the expression of everyday life, with the delusions but also the joys. The book deals with how the parents discover the disorder in their child, the feelings and fears it produced, and also how the children themselves can cope with it and how they feel about it.

To my knowledge, this is the first time families express themselves in detail and can express how the disorder is perceived "from the inside." Such an approach should prove most useful for the newly affected familes who are suddenly faced with a disorder they had never heard of and who discover that their child has this mysterious disease.

Olivier Dulac, Epilepsia

Thank you so very much for your latest *Brainstorms* book. I have just finished reading it and I must tell you that I felt every emotion imaginable. Some of those children seemed to have a better grasp of their situation than I have. I cried, I laughed, and experienced all the feelings in between. The parents' stories were truly heartbreaking. To watch your child go through everything that epilepsy brings with it must be a horrifying thing. Most told their stories in such a realistic way that I had a mental image of just what they were going through.

A Reader

THE BRAINSTORMS HEALER
EPILEPSY IN OUR EXPERIENCE

*Stories of Health Care Professionals as
Care Providers and Patients*

Steven C. Schachter, M.D.
*Comprehensive Epilepsy Center
Beth Israel Deaconess Medical Center;
Harvard Medical School
Boston, Massachusetts*

A. James Rowan, M.D.
*Department of Neurology
Mount Sinai School of Medicine;
Neurology Service
Bronx VA Medical Service
New York, New York*

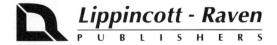
Lippincott - Raven
P U B L I S H E R S

Printed in the United States of America

ISBN 0-781-71688-8

Care has been taken to confirm the accuracy of the information presented and to describe generally accepted practices. However, the authors, editors, and publisher are not responsible for errors or omission or for any consequences from application of the information in this book and make no warranty, express or implied, with respect to the contents of the publication.

The authors, editors and publisher have exerted every effort to ensure that drug selection and dosage set forth in this text are in accordance with current recommendations and practice at the time of publication. However, in view of ongoing research, changes in government regulations, and the constant flow of information relating to drug therapy and drug reactions, the reader is urged to check the package insert for each drug for any change in indications and dosage and for added warnings and precautions. This is particularly important when the recommended agent is a new or infrequently employed drug.

Some drugs and medical devices presented in this publication have Food and Drug Administration (FDA) clearance for limited use in restricted research settings. It is the responsibility of the health care provider to ascertain the FDA status of each drug or device planned for use in their clinical practice.

9 8 7 6 5 4 3 2 1

Dedication

This book is dedicated to the memory of J. Kiffin Penry, M.D.

CONTENTS

PREFACE

The Brainstorms Healer: Epilepsy in Our Experience is the fourth in a series of books about the personal aspects of seizures and epilepsy. The first book, *Brainstorms: Epilepsy in Our Words* (Raven Press, 1993), contained many first-person accounts of adults with epilepsy. The second book, *The Brainstorms Companion: Epilepsy in Our View* (Raven Press, 1995), provided the perspectives of family members and friends of adults with seizures as well as guidelines for living safely with seizures. The third book, *The Brainstorms Family: Epilepsy on Our Terms* (Lippincott–Raven Publishers, 1996), consisted of stories by children with seizures and by their parents, as well as a glossary of medical terms and guidelines for schoolteachers.

Soon after the publication of *Brainstorms: Epilepsy in Our Words*, I was pleased to find that colleagues all around the world understood and appreciated its intent and mission. I was particularly gratified that they had read the book themselves, in addition to making it available to their patients. Many of these physicians and nurses shared their own personal experiences with me.

I was further amazed by the many health-care professionals who approached me at medical conferences or called to introduce themselves and to personally thank me, in confidence, for *Brainstorms: Epilepsy in Our Words* because it helped them to cope with *their own* epilepsy.

It appeared to me that stories of health care providers who care for patients with epilepsy, as well as personal accounts of health-care providers *who themselves have* epilepsy, would add two important and integral perspectives to the *Brainstorms* series. Several conversations with my close friend and co-editor, Jim Rowan, M.D., and with long-time supporter Cynthia Joyce, then with CIBA-Geigy, reinforced this belief and gave me the encouragement to proceed. Therefore, Dr. Rowan and I invited professionals with a variety of different perspectives on epilepsy—physicians, nurses, social workers, neuropsychologists, therapists, electroencephalography technologists, and physicians' secretaries—to reflect on their experiences. Some have worked for decades with patients who have epilepsy or have lived with their own seizures for years. Others have only begun to live with their own seizures or to treat epilepsy. Their stories have all been assembled in this book. Many other wonderful professionals were unable to participate because of schedule constraints.

The primary purpose of this book is to present the perspectives of health-care professionals from around the world as they describe their daily efforts to help patients with epilepsy or discuss their ongoing struggles with their own seizures. It is intended for anyone who interacts with epilepsy patients on a professional level. Readers will have an opportunity to evaluate their own feelings and reactions to their daily encounters with patients. It is also hoped that patients and their families will read this book and better understand what their doctors, nurses, and other health-care providers experience in their practices and feel in their hearts—their emotional highs and lows, their successes, and their failures. We hope that these insights will strengthen communication and increase understanding between patients with epilepsy and the professionals who care for them.

The volume begins with a tribute by Dr. Rowan to the late Kiffin Penry, M.D. In many ways, Dr. Penry embodied what the *Brainstorms* books seek to achieve. The book is then divided into two sections. The first section consists of stories about their patients by an international group of professionals, whose names are listed in the Appendix. The second section contains personal stories by providers with epilepsy. Their professional backgrounds are identified at the beginning of their passages, but their names will remain anonymous.

The Brainstorms Healer: Epilepsy in Our Experience reveals the wide range of emotions experienced by those who work with epilepsy patients and their families—the frustration of failing to control seizures, the inspiration of patients who persevere despite all odds, the sadness of losing a patient, the gratitude toward patients who bring meaning into the lives of their care providers, and the elation of enabling patients to live up to their potential.

We are all born with a soul and the potential to develop that soul for the betterment of us all. The special people who share their experiences in this book are among those who have done just that, even when challenged by personal hardships, emotional setbacks, and physical disabilities. I am proud to call them my friends and colleagues. Each time I read their words I gain renewed strength, encouragement, and commitment to my patients and the epilepsy movement.

This book also records, for the first time, the profound, uplifting, and often heartbreaking experiences of practitioners with seizures who come to understand first-hand the perspective of patients with epilepsy. As in the other *Brainstorms* books, the words of the contributors with seizures portray the finest representations of the human spirit—people whose courage and sustained commitment enable them to lead meaningful lives despite monumental obstacles. Each of the contributors has my profound thanks and deepest admiration.

Alan Krumholz, M.D., former Chair of the Professional Advisory Board (PAB) of the Epilepsy Foundation of America, was helpful in contacting PAB members and inviting their contributions for this book. I would like to thank Dr. Brien J. Smith for courageously accepting my invitation to write a foreword on behalf of the providers with epilepsy and Dr. B. J. Wilder for writing the foreword from the perspective of a clinician. My special thanks go to Cecile Davis for her hard work and persistent diligence throughout this project. I would like to acknowledge the enthusiastic support of Lippincott–Raven Healthcare. Thanks to Cathy Somer for her excellent editorial assistance. Finally, I would like to praise Sherry Shaw-Pickle and Novartis Pharmaceuticals Corporation for their continued support of the *Brainstorms* series and their distribution of this book and its three predecessors.

I invite those who would like to share their own stories or their reactions to this book to write to me in care of Comprehensive Epilepsy Center, Beth Israel Deaconess Medical Center, East Campus, 330 Brookline Avenue, K-478, Boston, Massachusetts 02215.

Steven C. Schachter, M.D.
December 22, 1997

FOREWORD

I am honored to write this foreword to *The Brainstorms Healer: Epilepsy in Our Experience*. I hope that my experiences and those of some of my patients will be meaningful to the reader.

Epilepsy can be the most chronic of neurologic diseases. The patient's well-being can depend on the sometimes overused term *doctor–patient relationship*. How is this relationship established between the doctor and the patient with epilepsy? A favorite admonishment of one of my professors in medical school was, "Doctor, just listen to your patient. He will tell you not only what is wrong with him but also why he came to see you." Certainly, to establish the doctor–patient relationship that fosters the best long-term outcome requires listening.

I recently attended a weekend conference on epilepsy for neurology residents. The format was that of lectures, interactive discussions, and case presentations, with ample time for the faculty and residents to exchange ideas. One of the residents asked why I had become interested in epilepsy. Friends, students, patients, and colleagues have asked me this question on many occasions. However, having the question asked again gave me time to reflect on just why I have spent more than 30 years in this field.

After graduating from medical school in 1955, I served in the Army Medical Corps for several years and had the opportunity to set up and run an outpatient clinic for military dependents, in addition to carrying out the duties of a regimental surgeon (mainly administering sick call). The clinic was in a semiremote area of California, and wives and children had followed the regiment for a long period of specialized training. I became a family physician. I soon realized that listening to patients was essential. I completed my residency and entered private practice as a family doctor in a small, out-of-the-way community in northern Florida. I had the opportunity of providing for most of the medical needs and many of the psychological needs of my patients. Once more, my professor's statement about listening to the patient proved to be true.

Several years later I did a residency in neurology and a fellowship in epilepsy and neurophysiology. After joining the faculty at the University of Florida, I took on the Epilepsy Clinic. My immersion in epilepsy had begun. In many ways it was similar to being in a restricted family practice. By listening to each patient, I could not only arrive at a diagnosis and often localize the epileptic focus but gain insight into the patient's fears, needs, expectations, self-esteem and, importantly, what the patient expected of me. Listening to the patient encompasses more than tabulating how many seizures and drug side effects the patient has and how compliant the patient has been. The management of patients with epilepsy means becoming their family physician.

The physician deals not only with seizures and medications but with many of the patient's other medical problems and some of the patient's emotional ones. The patient wishes to be seizure-free, to drive an automobile, to be like everyone else, and to be in control of his or her own destiny. Unfortunately, epilepsy often prevents patients from achieving these goals. Patients with epilepsy expect physicians to do their best to manage their disorder, but patients need more than that. In the absence of therapeutic success, the expectation and need is that the physician will just be there for them. Patients want their doctor to listen. Many of my patients have expressed this need in different ways. One day in the clinic when I was feeling sorry for myself for not being able to help a patient with very refractory seizures obtain a better therapeutic response, the patient consoled me by saying, "Doctor, you've been here and you've listened to me. I can always count on you for that."

Listening sometimes means waiting for the real problem to emerge. At the end of her freshman year at the University of Florida, Mary, a very pretty patient of mine, informed me that she would not be returning to the university the next year. I had made the diagnosis of juvenile myoclonic epilepsy the previous September and had placed her on medication, and she had had no further seizures. I had considered her case a complete success. She was driving, had joined a sorority, was making good grades, and had a boyfriend. She had gained weight, and I did note she was wearing a dark, smock-type dress and seemed depressed. I waited and listened. After some time and tears, I realized she was devastated by what turned out to be significant weight gain, which had prompted the smock-like dress. She had decided not to return to college because of embarrassment and loss of self-esteem over her weight gain. We worked together and made a medication change, and Mary will soon be a senior.

I recall Ann, a 13-year-old whom I suspected of having psychogenic nonepileptic seizures. One day in clinic, after shooing her mother out of the examining room, I gave Ann the opportunity to talk to me alone, and in a short time she told me about being sexually abused. This revelation helped explain her psychogenic seizures and led to appropriate therapy and, I hope, to her recovery. Mrs. B. was a schoolteacher. She was the overly concerned and anxious mother of a 15-year-old epilepsy patient of mine who was small of stature. He was really doing quite well, free from seizures and drug side effects. Mrs. B. finally revealed her worry that her son would never grow any taller because of his epilepsy and the medications he was taking. Further inquiry revealed that the mother's father had been very short until a late growth spurt that began at age 16. A little bit of listening and reassuring aborted a planned, expensive course of growth hormone treatment reluctantly suggested by an endocrinologist. A year later, Mrs. B.'s son's own growth spurt began.

Sometimes, listening to teenagers can be informative. Nancy, a 16-year-old who had been my patient for a number of years, had particularly difficult-to-manage epilepsy. One day she came to clinic for her 6-month visit and informed me she had been seizure-free for almost 6 months. I was delighted, thinking that the last medication change and my skill in managing her case had finally succeeded. I asked her the particulars of our finally achieving success. She then informed me that after her last visit she had decided to start taking her medications. After all, it was time to get her driver's license. Even though her blood levels had been somewhat erratic, I had thought she was compliant. Nancy denied having been noncompliant but said that shortly before coming to her previous visits, she would always take a few capsules, anticipating that I might check her blood level. This was my lesson about epilepsy in the adolescent.

Listening to patients does more than improve patient care. It builds confidence and self-esteem. The patient loses dependence on the doctor and becomes a partner in the management of his or her epilepsy. A lasting rapport and real friendship develop. One of my patients, on going away to college, told me that he was really going to miss his visits because we had become such good friends.

Often, if the physician waits an extra minute or so, the patient will share his or her real concerns and fears with the doctor. Epilepsy can be a devastating disorder. Parental overprotection can render even seizure-free patients emotional cripples. The physician who spends time with patients and their families can help to prevent many pitfalls from occurring. The patient, the patient's family, and the physician are all amply rewarded with the outcome. The doctor's and the patient's quality of life are enhanced.

The changing medical scene has imposed a number of limitations on physicians and patients. Managed health care limits time and sets schedules for doctors and patients to follow. Patients may be allowed only one or a few visits to see their neurologist or epileptologist. In these difficult times, the *Brainstorms* books will help both patients and physicians share in and profit from the experiences of others.

B. J. Wilder, M.D.

FOREWORD

Epilepsy is a condition with protean manifestations. Even experts may have difficulty classifying certain types of seizures, epilepsies, and epilepsy syndromes. It is therefore not surprising that many physicians and other health-care workers have a limited understanding of seizures and a simplified view of epilepsy.

Even so, this problem is minor from the perspective of patients, who are more concerned about whether their doctor understands how they feel and what they are experiencing. Many physicians fail to spend enough time with their patients to enable them to freely convey their feelings, experiences, and questions. Issues that may appear trivial to physicians are often of great significance to patients. A doctor–patient relationship is therapeutically successful when the clinician is conscientious and open-minded *and* takes the time necessary to listen and respond appropriately to the patient's questions and concerns.

Health-care professionals share a common goal: to provide high-quality care to the sick and to prevent illness in healthy people through education, understanding, and compassion. Empathy for patients, particularly patients with epilepsy, is an integral and invaluable ingredient. However, for physicians and other professionals, identifying the emotional needs of patients with epilepsy can be challenging. The best approach to follow in attempting to establish a successful therapeutic alliance is to enter the relationship with an open mind and to *really listen* to the patient and his or her family.

The three sides of the therapeutic triangle are the patient, the family, and the health-care provider. The previous *Brainstorms* books, compiled by Steven Schachter, provided insights from two sides of the therapeutic triangle; this book completes it. This volume, *The Brainstorms Healer: Epilepsy in Our Experience*, presents the observations and feelings of epileptologists, epilepsy nurses, and other professionals about caring for patients with epilepsy. Contributors from around the world who strive to provide the highest level of care share their insights into the dynamics of epileptology and the profound impact their patients have had on their lives. These are caring professionals writing about extraordinary patients.

A portion of this book is reserved for the stories of a group of health-care professionals who also have epilepsy. Like the other stories, the perspectives of this unique group of people cannot be found in any major textbook on the topic. Each of these persons has viewed and experienced epilepsy as both patient and health-care provider. I belong to that group.

When I was first invited by Steve Schachter to write a foreword that conveyed my personal experiences with epilepsy, I had significant reservations. Like other patients with epilepsy, I tend to keep this fact about me submerged, not only because I view it as a private matter but because of my wariness about society's stereotypes of people with epilepsy.

For these reasons, in the early stages of my career I rarely discussed my condition with colleagues and patients. Then, ironically at a time when my principal activity at work was to evaluate patients with intractable seizures for possible epilepsy surgery, I had my first seizure in 15 years. Along with the disappointment of having a breakthrough seizure, I had physical pain from a fractured spine I sustained in the process. These problems seemed insignificant when I subsequently learned that I had a brain tumor.

In the following years, some patients who were undergoing presurgical evaluations became aware of my past experiences. Their reactions were extraordinary. Many were tremendously relieved when they found out that I had been "on both sides of the fence" and that I could truly relate to the issues and concerns that were bothering them. They felt comforted knowing that I could appreciate, at the deepest personal level, the many facets of their illness, their daily struggles, and their fears and hopes about epilepsy surgery.

My experiences throughout my own diagnostic evaluation, brain surgery, and recovery affected my outlook as patient—and as physician. They not only reaffirmed for me the importance of one-on-one doctor–patient communication but also convinced me that sharing my personal experiences with epilepsy could benefit other patients and physicians.

As major changes in health care descend on us, including ever-increasing demands to limit the time we spend with patients, we cannot forget the most important part of our daily work—talking and listening to our patients. After all, theirs are the stories we ultimately tell. Many of their stories are in this book. After reading them, we will better understand how patients with epilepsy affect our lives and we will learn not to underestimate how much we can positively affect theirs.

Brien J. Smith, M.D.

A TRIBUTE TO JAMES KIFFIN PENRY, M.D. (1929–1996)

Steve Schachter and I have dedicated this book to the late Kiffin Penry. In his memory, all of the royalties from this book will be donated to the Kiffin Penry Memorial Fund of the Epilepsy Foundation of America. I hope that the following tribute will convey my feelings for Kiffin and what he meant to the epilepsy movement.

Recognizing the desperate need for additional antiepileptic drugs but understanding that industry was unlikely to undertake the challenge alone, Kiffin established the Antiepileptic Drug Development Program (ADD), which systematically investigated hundreds of compounds, looking for the most promising to undergo development. At the same time he enlisted the cooperation of pharmaceutical firms, convincing them of the pressing need for new drugs and the important benefits of developing compounds that would attack epilepsy at fundamental mechanistic levels. The fruits of this enormous effort are visible today, for the number of effective antiepileptic drugs has doubled and more are on the way. The lives of hundreds of thousands of patients have been directly affected by this signal achievement. But there was more—much more.

A major milestone in the history of epilepsy in the United States was the authorization by Congress in 1974 of the Commission for the Control of Epilepsy and Its Consequences. At the time, the United States lagged behind many other countries in providing a broad spectrum of services for people with epilepsy. No centers comparable to the established programs in, for example, the Netherlands or Norway existed in the United States. Moreover, research efforts in the United States lacked focus and appeared to be divorced from clinical activities. As head of the Epilepsy Branch, Kiffin led the effort to implement the recommendations of the Commission, which included as a centerpiece the establishment in the United States of comprehensive centers for diagnosis, treatment, and research in the field of epilepsy. Under Kiffin's prescient guidance, three comprehensive epilepsy centers were established, changing forever the practice of epileptology in this country. Now, a scant 25 years later, scores of comprehensive epilepsy centers dot the landscape, offering hope to thousands of patients and underlying a substantial increase in research productivity.

These major achievements, however, give an incomplete measure of the man. Today the epilepsy community enjoys enormous contributions from scores of clinical and research epileptologists nurtured, trained, and inspired by Kiffin, who keep his spirit alive. Although Kiffin reached the pinnacle of epileptology-related affairs in the United States and internationally, he never lost his concern for individual patients. He understood their suffering and was determined to change their lives for the better. Anyone who had the good fortune to engage in late-night chats with Kiffin—for example, during his outstanding Minifellowship Program—understood his compassion, dedication, and humanity. Although we are the poorer for his loss, his students and their accomplishments, both now and in the future, will bear enduring testament to his life's achievements.

When the fight against epilepsy is won, as it surely will be, Kiffin's contributions to the victory will never be forgotten. This is a fitting memorial to a singular life.

A. James Rowan, M.D.

CONTRIBUTORS

Steven C. Schachter, M.D. *Director of Clinical Research, Comprehensive Epilepsy Center, Beth Israel Deaconess Medical Center; Associate Professor of Neurology, Harvard Medical School, Boston, Massachusetts*

A. James Rowan, M.D. *Professor and Vice-Chairman, Department of Neurology, Mount Sinai School of Medicine; Chief, Neurology Service, Bronx VA Medical Service, New York, New York*

Brien J. Smith, M.D. *Director, Epilepsy Monitoring Unit, Henry Ford Health System, Detroit, Michigan*

B. J. Wilder, M.D. *Professor Emeritus, Department of Neurology, University of Florida College of Medicine, Gainesville, Florida*

Descriptions by Providers

❖ ❖ ❖ ❖ ❖

1

In my 30 years of working with epilepsy patients and their families, I have come into contact with thousands of people in a variety of ways. My career began in Montreal. From there I went to the West Coast, then to the East Coast, and finally to the Midwest. Several of my former patients have followed my career moves across the country. They continue to send Christmas cards, call to say they are still seizure-free, and tell me how much they appreciate the part I played in changing their lives. I have learned that some of my patients divorced their spouses after becoming seizure-free. Their family dynamics changed so much that it was really better for them to start a new life. Ironically, my commitment to patients with epilepsy most certainly contributed to my divorce from my first husband.

I'm sure I have felt every human emotion at some time concerning one patient or another. Every time I believe I am done with this manuscript I think of someone else who made me laugh or cry. My career has sustained me through personal triumphs and personal tragedies. It has also afforded me the opportunity to work with some of the most intelligent, caring, and wonderful people in the world.

People with epilepsy are all different in some ways, yet in other ways they have many things in common. Let me share with you several stories.

The emergency room (ER) staff knew Mr. C very well. When he was seen there after a seizure, they used to send him directly to my office. One morning he arrived via the ER with a sheepish grin on his face and said, "I was in the grocery store—the peanut butter and jam section, I guess." I knew immediately that he was right—he was covered from head to foot with peanut butter and jam.

Mrs. G had infrequent complex partial seizures. One night, while cooking dinner for her family, she had a seizure. She dropped the ladle and continued to stir the boiling soup with her hand. The paramedics called me to ask what to do for the seizure, apparently oblivious of her hand injury!

Mr. D was a noncompliant and rebellious but very bright young man who did not do well participating in group classes about epilepsy. He did, however, listen during one-on-one counseling and learned about his seizures. He eventually became compliant, realized his seizures were not his whole life, and turned into someone he was proud to be.

I have seen many children who have hundreds of seizures every day. Some children with epilepsia partialis continua for whom I have cared underwent hemispherectomies. At their follow-up visits, I could see how each child was progressing toward reaching his or her full potential. Some children made amazing strides in just a few months.

One of the most frustrating situations I encounter time and time again is overprotection by parents of a child with epilepsy. In my own life, I have been blessed with four healthy children. I do not know how *I* would handle having a child with seizures. However, parents of severely handicapped children often cope very well, whereas parents of minimally affected children sometimes cannot cope at all. In particular, I recall a nurse whose 10-year-old son had a febrile seizure at the age of 18 months. After that, every time he twitched or jerked in his sleep she thought he was seizing. He underwent EEG monitoring twice for epilepsy and once for a sleep disorder. When his mother found out that the results of each test were totally normal, she was dissatisfied and asked me if her son could have depth electrodes. She had read that some seizures can be missed when scalp EEG electrodes are used to monitor for seizures.

I can think of two children who, although their seizures are controlled by medications, have *never* been to school on a regular basis because the parents, in both cases, are afraid that their children will have seizures there—one child is 10 years old and the other is 14.

Of course, all of us who care for patients with epilepsy run into awkward situations. These can be difficult to categorize. We are simply relieved when the patient leaves the office or the hospital and goes home. I remember a homosexual patient who was admitted to the hospital for video/EEG monitoring with implanted electrodes. While he was being monitored, he tried to maintain sexual relations with his very emotional partner. Then there was another young man with implanted electrodes whom I was assisting to the bathroom. He had a generalized seizure in the bathroom, and the cable that connected the electrode wires to the wall became tangled in the intravenous pole. While I was protecting his head from banging against the commode, several of the electrode wires snapped. Then there was the girlfriend of another patient who always seemed to be blocking the camera while her boyfriend (the patient) was having complex partial seizures.

It is often difficult for medical students to get used to being on video when they examine a patient who is undergoing EEG monitoring. One such student forgot he was on camera when he witnessed what he thought was a pseudoseizure. He thought the patient was malingering, slapped him across the face, and commanded, "Snap out of it!"

Many of us have encountered patients who go through the first week of EEG monitoring without having any seizures. We then ask them if there is anything that will precipitate a seizure. Some patients reply that nothing will trigger their seizures and others say the usual, such as skipping medications. Then there was the man who said, "A six-pack of beer and sex will do it every time."

Frightening incidents that are quite unexpected sometimes occur. I remember one young woman who had relatively infrequent seizures. When she had a prolonged seizure in the monitoring unit, she became frankly psychotic and was sure she was the devil. On reflection, some incidents are rather funny. I remember one young woman who had a complex partial seizure while a doctor was visiting her. During her postictal confusion she grabbed his necktie and would not let go. The bluer his face got, the tighter she held on. Eventually she let go and everything was fine.

Wada tests can be very exciting to do. Mr. P became rather euphoric when amytal was injected into his right carotid artery. As he tried to jump off the table, he exclaimed, "This is better than sex!" Mr. L was a wealthy, upper-class man from India who had been educated at Oxford and spoke English better than most of us. Sadly, this man had traveled around the world trying to persuade someone to consider him for epilepsy surgery. Although he had only a few seizures each year, this was unacceptable to him in light of his social status in India. When his dominant cerebral hemisphere was injected with amytal, he momentarily stopped speaking. When he began to talk, it was only in Hindu. After he completed the presurgical evaluation, he underwent epilepsy surgery and became seizure-free. Tragically, he died of a heart attack 3 years later.

Father M was one of my favorite patients. He began to have complex partial seizures after being kicked in the head during a high school game of water polo. He had tremendous will and motivation to open all doors that were closed to him because of his epilepsy. He was told that he could not become a priest if he had seizures—but he did. He was told that he could not become a teacher in a Catholic school if he had seizures—but, again, he did. At the beginning of each school year he told his students that he was not perfect. No one was perfect, he taught them. He would then proceed to describe his seizures to his students and explain what to do if he had one. He never received anything but praise from his students and their parents.

Father M was told he would never be admitted to a top law school if he had seizures; yet the day before his seizure surgery he was accepted to Harvard Law School. He had a wonderful sense of humor and became acquainted with many of the other patients during his hospitalizations. In those days, patients could stay in the hospital for weeks at a time undergoing various tests. Father M claimed not to know how to play cards but regularly beat nurses and patients at poker. While filling out a routine psychological paper-and-pencil test (the MMPI), he called me into his room and asked if he could skip a question. I told Father M that he needed to answer every question to the best of his ability and asked him which question was troubling him. "Is your sex life satisfactory?" he said.

2

Despite the many advances in the treatment of epilepsy, many patients still have seizures, sometimes with no decrease in their frequency or severity. That is why I am impressed that most of my patients still maintain a lust for life, show great courage, and continue to focus on the positive aspects of their lives.

Two of the most important problems faced by people with epilepsy are loneliness and difficulty finding a job. Consequently, social rehabilitation programs have a very important role in their overall treatment plan. Unfortunately, however, most physicians who work in the field of neurorehabilitation have no training in epilepsy, and most books on neurorehabilitation do not include chapters on epilepsy.

As a doctor and an epileptologist, I experience the deepest frustration when I am notified of the sudden and unexpected death of one of my patients. Often these patients have been found dead in bed, lying dead on the floor of their apartment, or drowned in the bathtub. They are invariably young and are often at the beginning of their lives. I never forget them, and I feel that I have truly and ultimately failed them.

Sudden death among patients with epilepsy is something we do not discuss with patients often enough. But how should this issue be addressed? Should we tell every patient with epilepsy about the risk? Most of all, should more research be done to find out why this happens and how to prevent it?

Recently, a lovely 24-year-old woman with epilepsy was found dead in the bathtub. Only a month before she had proudly shown me her 18-month-old daughter and described how she had succeeded in finding a nice apartment. She was optimistic because she felt as if she were starting a new life (her boyfriend had left her when she became pregnant). I often think of her daughter and wonder who is taking care of her now.

Another one of my young patients, a 25-year-old man, died last year while in bed. His parents had encouraged him to live alone so that his life would be as normal as possible. They had visited him that evening and had eaten dinner with him. He had a girlfriend, but she had not been there that night.

The next morning he was found lying face down on his bed, fully dressed. No one was sure whether or not he had experienced a seizure. When his parents called me, we talked about the problem of sudden death and epilepsy. They wondered why his other doctors and I had not told them or their son that this could occur. I asked them if they thought he would have lived any differently if he had known. If we told every patient with epilepsy about this possibility, some might not dare live independent lives or might be burdened by anxiety, knowing that they might not awake in the morning.

To this day, I do not know if my answer was appropriate.

3

During the many years I worked as a surgical nurse, I occasionally took care of patients with a history of seizures, usually grand mal seizures. I can remember being worried about their safety during seizures and trying to protect them from injury. I also remember being concerned during their postictal periods because they needed to be reoriented and to be monitored for other medical or surgical problems.

However, these experiences didn't really prepare me for what I encountered when I began to work more closely with seizure patients as part of a team researching a new antiepileptic drug. This was an inpatient study in which EEG monitoring and closed-circuit television were used. I was unfamiliar with the technology, but the range of seizure types that these patients had was even more unfamiliar to me.

I was not prepared to manage some of the unusual seizure behaviors that occurred as we began to take these patients off their seizure medications for the study. For example, we admitted a patient who typically wandered during his seizures and would become hostile when he was restrained. When I witnessed the beginning stages of one of his seizures, I was terrified because I could not predict what was going to happen next.

The patient ran out of the room with the EEG monitoring equipment still connecting him to the wall. When an observer tried to restrain him, he reacted physically with a wild look in his eyes. I knew enough to say to let him go and asked everyone else not to touch or restrain him. I quickly disconnected the electrode wires from the wall before he broke anything, while at the same time trying not to touch or aggravate him. As he ran down the hallway, my thoughts concerned his safety, the safety of other nearby personnel, and my responsibility to monitor his seizure activity for the study. I still didn't know what to expect. I stayed with him, talked to him, and tried to redirect him. I had no idea how long this would last, how far I would have to follow him, or what I could do to protect him. Would he try to hurt me?

Suddenly, the patient turned around and returned to the research unit and tried to open a locked door. That scared me. Was he going to break the door down or, worse, hurt himself? Then, when he lay down in the middle of the hallway, I breathed a sigh of relief and thought that now he would be unresponsive with postictal confusion. I tried to administer intravenous seizure medication, but to my surprise he awoke and looked at me wildly. I was fearful of him because I thought he might misunderstand my intentions and hurt me. As his nurse, I felt helpless during this phase of his seizure. To me, this patient's seizures were more dramatic, frightening, and unpredictable than any of the grand mal seizures I had ever witnessed. Fortunately, the patient did eventually become postictal.

Since then, I have been very conscious of patient safety at all times. I worry that I can't always protect patients from harm while they are hospitalized, even with all the precautions that are taken.

The first instance in which a patient injured himself in my presence (while I was observing his seizure) took me completely by surprise. When the seizure began, the patient was in a chair next to the bed. He stared and became unresponsive. At this point he was still connected to the EEG monitoring equipment and I was waiting for him to become alert enough for me to assist him into bed. I knew not to touch him because in the postictal state he, too, could act in a hostile manner. So I only stood there and observed him. And waited. Then, without any warning, he catapulted forward off the chair head first and hit his forehead on the hard floor! This happened so quickly that I couldn't help or protect him. The next thing I saw was that he was in the midst of a grand mal seizure. Other staff nurses helped me pad the floor under him until the convulsing stopped. His face turned blue and then the seizure seemed to end.

All this seemed to last an eternity but actually went on for only 2 to 4 minutes. I felt helpless because there wasn't much that I could do, and terrible because my patient had hit his head and I couldn't have prevented it. I was worried that he had suffered a skull fracture from hitting the floor so hard. I applied and held ice to his forehead while he was postictal and unresponsive, and saw that he had also bitten his tongue. Later, when he was alert, I discussed the seizure with him. I was struck by his calm attitude about the whole thing. What amazed me even more was that he said his head didn't hurt that much. That made me feel better, especially after it became clear that his injury was not serious.

Why do I find some seizures frightening? I think it has to do with not being able to control the situation or anticipate what will happen next, along with being unable to completely protect the patient from injury. That uncertainty is unsettling for me and also, I suspect, for other people who observe seizures.

4

Of all the medical conditions that I treat as a neurologist, epilepsy is the most special. My interest in epilepsy is very close to my interest in civil rights. Because I am a member of a minority group, I can identify with epilepsy patients. Patients with seizures have historically been misunderstood, discriminated against, abused, and even punished for circumstances beyond their control.

Although humans may think of themselves as more socially enlightened than animals, the unfortunate reality is that we often lower ourselves to the same level as farm chickens. Discrimination is nothing more than the human expression of the pecking order. Just as chickens peck at one another, the weakest chicken being at the bottom of the pyramid, so can people with seizures find themselves outcast from society by those who are "civilized."

People with epilepsy are often in the same drifting boat as many blacks, Hispanics, women, gays, and members of other minority groups. Anyone who is different or misunderstood is often abused.

Indeed, epilepsy patients have been more than discriminated against. As we know, it was acceptable in the past to burn a person with epilepsy at the stake because it was believed that he or she was possessed by demons.

There is always some false justification for discrimination. In the case of epilepsy, a number of myths about persons with epilepsy have permeated our society for centuries. An especially popular one is that the person with seizures is possessed. These myths have survived in order to explain aspects of seizures such as falling to the ground, foaming at the mouth, jerking, confusion, and agitation. The root of discrimination is often fear and lack of public education. Seizures often elicit fear of the unknown in observers.

Just mentioning the word *epilepsy* for the first time to patients and their families causes a change in their facial expressions that reveals *their* fear and lack of knowledge about the condition. I often think about how challenging it is to educate them, when centuries of oral and written tradition, including sacred books such as the Bible, make reference to demonic possession or the inferior mind of the epileptic.

I, too, have been discriminated against, simply because I am Hispanic. My language, accent, culture, and way of thinking are different from those of mainstream Americans. But at least I can go back to my own country, in which I am just like everyone else. This is impossible for people with epilepsy. Where can they go? They will always have their seizures to bear. That is why I attempt to treat epilepsy patients with the dignity and respect that every human being deserves, regardless of any characteristics that make them different from others. I hope that other physicians will do the same.

5

I entered the atmosphere of a hospital-based epilepsy center straight from the sterile isolation of a chemistry laboratory. At the center, which was both a monitoring unit and an outpatient clinic, the most important dictum was, "Listen to patients and their families." I heeded that advice and was deeply impressed by the involvement of families in the lives of their family members with intractable epilepsy. What I learned was more than empathy or compassion—I learned about the impact of epilepsy on caregivers, parents, siblings, and spouses, and about the many ways in which people cope with problems, accommodate themselves to circumstances, and deal with guilt or frustration.

Of course, these lessons can be extrapolated to other chronic medical disorders. My exposure to patients and their families in the epilepsy center has helped me as I have faced illness myself and in my family.

The key elements in coping with illness can be summarized as: Don't give in, and don't just bemoan your plight. Learn how to outsmart the circumstances that seem to hold you back. Spend your energies developing coping strategies that allow you both to accommodate to your situation and to maximize your potential.

The family of a boy whose epilepsy was hopelessly uncontrolled made every effort to carry on a relatively normal lifestyle. We heard from them only when his seizures went on for days without ceasing. His mother once told me that she made the decision to come to the center only when her washing machine overheated from too many loads of sheets that had become soiled from her son's seizure-induced incontinence. Now, that's coping!

6

I have been a nurse for many years, but my experience in caring for patients with epilepsy was very limited until I became involved in research protocols for investigating new drug treatments for uncontrolled seizures. Watching the seizures was frightening and a little overwhelming in the beginning. Seizures were so different from one patient to the next! Initially, I think it was the uncertainty about when they would occur that made them so scary. Seizures were so unpredictable. Some patients had no warning that a seizure was about to occur and, even worse, no memory of the seizure after it was over.

I was disconcerted because, when a patient's seizure began, I would not know in advance what it would be like and how long it would last. I learned from experience that a seizure could be as mild as a strange sensation, a rush through the body, a quick staring spell, or a change in consciousness accompanied by facial grimacing and extremity movements. Or, it could be as dramatic as a generalized seizure, in which violent movements of the legs and arms occurred accompanied by guttural sounds from the throat, cyanosis, and loss of bladder control. Some seizures lasted only a few seconds, whereas others went on for minutes. When a seizure began, I had no idea how I would have to react.

I am now more comfortable and confident when I observe seizures. Yet even after all these months of frequent exposure to seizure activity, I still get a rush of adrenaline once a patient starts to have a seizure. Simple and complex partial seizures are usually very manageable, but I still never know if one will secondarily generalize. My main goal, always, is to keep the patient safe from injury and to observe closely so I that can report the event with accuracy.

It is often painful to watch a patient with a generalized seizure experience such uncontrolled, intense and violent gyrations. As I respond by positioning the patient and intervening in whatever ways are necessary to protect him or her from injury, I always silently pray that the seizure will end. I breathe a sigh of relief when the movements stop and all is quiet again.

I know that I can have absolutely no idea what it must be like to have a seizure. I can't help wondering why and how everything that we take for granted in our lives can suddenly get so scrambled and cause such chaos. I can only imagine how frightening it must be. I cannot even imagine the sensations and feelings a patient must have when emerging from a seizure: to have no idea what has happened, to be dazed or to feel confused, and to feel embarrassed about his or her behavior during the seizure. One of my patients can tell when he is postictal: "I know I have had a seizure because people are around me, staring, and they have that terrified look on their faces." Because of that remark, when I am caring for patients in the postictal period I always try to keep my voice soft and calm and my expression serene, while assuring them that they are safe and gradually reorienting them.

Because of my experiences, I can appreciate the enormously disruptive effect that epilepsy can have on all aspects of a person's life. One example is driving. Although I believe that driving restrictions are completely understandable and are often necessary to protect the safety of patients and others, I cannot imagine what it would be like not to be allowed to drive. This curtailment of personal freedom can in itself be truly distressing, not to mention the limitations it places on choices of where to live, work, and shop.

I have also come to realize that there is usually a lack of support and understanding in the community and the workplace for people with epilepsy, depending on the severity of their seizures. Furthermore, personal and family relations often become strained, and unbelievable things can happen. I still remember how horrified I was when one of my patients described how he was repeatedly robbed during his seizures while he was unconscious; his wallet, money, jewelry and clothing, and even his medical alert bracelet were each stolen at different times. What an outrage!

My overall experience in caring for patients with epilepsy has been decidedly positive. I have relished the opportunity to learn about epilepsy and have gained tremendous respect and admiration for people with seizures. In addition to having a better understanding of epilepsy, I am now far more sensitive and compassionate toward those who have seizures, and I have a greater appreciation for the profound impact that living with seizures has on their lives.

7

The following story is about a young man whose epilepsy could have been adequately treated by someone in the medical profession. However, nobody in that profession took an interest in his problems. That very indifference may have cost him his life.

I saw this patient in my private clinic after a referral from his general practitioner. In fact, it was the patient's parents who had finally persuaded their son to obtain a second opinion. He was only 27 years old, although he looked much older. He had suffered from epilepsy since he was 5 years old, when he had contracted encephalitis. He appeared frustrated and resigned. He felt there was nothing to live for and spoke in a strange, detached way, as if he had told his story so many times that he was tired of repeating it. And I am sure that he *had* repeated his story many times, because he was seen by a new physician every time he went to the epilepsy clinic.

The young man had attended the epilepsy clinic over a period of years, but his seizures could not be controlled with the available drugs. For the past several years he had been seen only annually. It was evident that the staff had given up on him. He was treated with a single antiepileptic drug, and the dosage was rarely changed. His records noted that although he still had many seizures, his seizure drug plasma level was within the therapeutic range. His blood level was the focus of the medical attention, not his seizures or overall well-being!

The patient lived alone. His hobby was to referee football (soccer) matches (he had previously played football himself). He seemed to have very few friends, if any, and often visited his elderly parents. He told me that his seizures—and he had many of them—affected his consciousness for a couple of minutes. He could not recall any part of his seizures. It had been that way for many years. He often did strange things during seizures. When refereeing a football match, he sometimes suddenly left the field during a seizure. He would walk through the clubhouse to his home without remembering that he was supposed to be refereeing the match. Occasionally, on his way home, he would stop at a tree and void, which he would never dream of doing normally.

He bicycled to work every day and often hit a tree or a wall along the way because of a seizure. He would then arrive at his job with bloody wounds on his face, unable to explain what had happened. It was clear to him that his friends often suspected him of being drunk, and he therefore isolated himself from others at work. Once he had a seizure at work, and when he regained consciousness he was standing with an electric drill in his mouth, biting down. Luckily, the current was switched off. Yet despite the attitudes of his co-workers, he was proud that he was able to keep his job as an electrical engineer.

I must admit that as I talked with him I became afraid of what might happen to him and considered ordering sick leave for him. At the same time, however, I realized that this might be the last time I would see him, because I knew that he would not accept my attempt to intervene in his life and impose restrictions on his lifestyle.

He told me that he had eight complex partial seizures per month, many of them with automatisms. Just before we finished our first appointment, he experienced such a seizure, as if he wanted to emphasize how many seizures he had. He suddenly lost full consciousness and started to look around with an expression full of fear. He made strange sounds, as though he were imitating a wounded animal. At the same time, he fumbled with all the things on my desk. His face grew pale and then red.

The seizure lasted only 2 minutes, although it seemed much longer to me. (Many patients' relatives say the same thing.) It took him about 20 minutes to become fully reoriented. Afterwards, he had no idea that he had just had a seizure, which indicated that he might actually be having many more seizures than he realized.

I explained to him that I had to obtain his records from the other hospitals and clinics that he had attended. My plan was to check his previous drug treatments before planning therapy for him. I was hopeful that I could improve his situation with some of the new drugs that he had never tried. I told him that if these new medications did not work I would consider him for surgery. Our National Health Board demands that all drugs be tried before surgery is considered.

It turned out that there were five drugs the patient had never tried. After prescribing trials of these drugs I saw him frequently in the outpatient clinic to find out if any of these medications had helped him. Unfortunately, none of the drugs had any effect on his seizures. We discussed the surgical program in detail. I was pleased when he told me that, without doubt, he immediately wanted to start the diagnostic process toward possible epilepsy surgery. He could not continue to accept life with so many seizures.

In my country, presurgical investigations are often done in the outpatient clinic, without the patient being required to be admitted to the hospital except for video/EEG monitoring of seizures. However, because there is a long waiting list for some of the tests, it may take up to 6 months to finish the workup. It is terribly stressful for patients to wait that long for all the tests to be completed. Unfortunately, the medical resources are poor in my region and epilepsy is not considered a high priority.

Given these constraints, we started the long process of determining whether the patient's epileptic focus was localized to a restricted, surgically accessible area of his brain. However, it soon became apparent that he often missed the scheduled tests without being able to explain why he did not show up. I thought that he might have forgotten his appointments because of seizures. Then he stopped coming altogether. I soon found out why.

I received the patient's death certificate from our medicolegal institute. While riding his bicycle to work, he had suddenly turned in front of a bus, presumably during a seizure. He had broken a number of bones and sustained major, fatal trauma to his inner organs. His aorta had been pulled apart.

I was shocked and depressed. Could my patient's death have been avoided? Should we have scheduled the tests more quickly? Should I have admitted him to the hospital for the tests? I knew that it was not rare for epilepsy patients to die suddenly and unexpectedly while waiting for surgery. I could have seen this patient much sooner in my clinic had he been referred a long time ago. Why did it take so many years to find out that he suffered from drug-resistant epilepsy? Although patients must assume responsibility for their own lives, show initiative, and not accept poor treatment, I still felt guilty.

This tragedy and other somewhat similar experiences have convinced me that providing accurate information about epilepsy to patients, relatives, and the population in general is very important.

If *you* have epilepsy, do not blindly trust your own doctor or the specialist in your hospital. Get a second opinion if your seizures cannot be controlled. Other drugs or approaches may be effective, including surgery. I try not to feel offended when my patients say that they want to see another doctor. Everyone with epilepsy deserves to receive the best possible treatment.

Conscientious medical care saves lives.

8

I remember a 30-year-old math teacher who had complex partial seizures. He was considerably distressed by his seizures, which occasionally embarrassed him in front of his class at school. His seizures did not respond to trials of the usual medications, and he went through a presurgical evaluation. To our surprise, his seizure focus turned out to be in the left temporal lobe, despite the fact that he had good mathematical and verbal abilities. He underwent a partial left anterior temporal lobectomy.

Unfortunately, the patient suffered a serious postoperative complication, one that was rare in my experience. A left posterior temporal hematoma developed at the margin of the resection, extending into Wernicke's area. Consequently, the man became profoundly aphasic. In addition, his complex partial seizures persisted.

The members of the medical care team, including me, were devastated by the complication, as was the patient. Nevertheless, he threw himself fully into his rehabilitation and his speech improved substantially. He moved to the South, where, he said, "people talk slow anyway." He gave up teaching mathematics because he lost most of his mathematical and computational skills. He earned an income by selling insurance.

One year after the man's surgery he returned to our institution because he was still having seizures. Naturally, we were reluctant to attempt any invasive procedures, but at the patient's request we put aside our distress over the previous complication. We felt obligated to see if anything could be done to help him, so we began by reviewing his current symptoms and then proceeded to EEG monitoring. Testing showed that his seizures were originating from remnants of the left posterior hippocampal area. After much intense discussion and the patient's extensive encouragement of the medical team (sometimes such encouragement flows in the reverse direction), we reoperated. This time the patient had no complications. Later, he went back to the South to live.

Three years later, our follow-up indicates that the patient is seizure-free and leads a full and independent life. His aphasia is not evident in casual conversation. He believes that his medical experience overall was extremely worthwhile and says that he would do it again in a moment.

I had a similar experience with an 8-year-old boy. He had cortical developmental anomalies that gave rise to a catastrophic seizure syndrome. He underwent surgery on his left frontal lobe at another institution, which resulted in postoperative hemorrhage and no improvement at all in his seizures. His parents had educated themselves about epilepsy and its treatment to a degree unusual even for the parents of severely challenged children, who often know more about epilepsy than their doctors do.

The child's parents wanted us to take another look at him. We therefore implanted a subdural grid over the left frontal region. The grid showed his seizure focus to be in the left premotor area, approximately 1 to 2 centimeters anterior to the primary motor cortex. Because their child had recurrent status epilepticus and had required medication doses high enough to cause major behavioral problems, his parents and the medical care team decided to perform another resection.

When he awakened from surgery, the child was densely hemiparetic on the right side. Although some degree of postoperative weakness had been expected, a dense hemiparesis had not. Again, the medical team lost considerable sleep over the complication and spent a very difficult week hoping that the boy's strength would return and that the seizures would not. After about a week the child began to show some return of tone in his right leg, and by the end of the following week he was able to walk independently with a limp. From that point on, further recovery proceeded rapidly.

Two years later the boy appears almost normal. He is seizure-free and off antiepileptic medications. His prognosis for continued seizure control appears good; the pathology report showed dysplastic cortex that did not extend beyond the margins of resection. This diseased tissue was undetectable on the magnetic resonance imaging scan of his brain, even on retrospective review.

These two episodes have taught me that seizure surgery, particularly high-risk procedures, can be a roller coaster for patients and families, as well as for the medical care team. In such situations we have to be cautious and to balance the risks dispassionately.

Although we must try to empathize with our patients, we cannot let our emotions interfere with our decision-making. Sometimes, when the situation looks darkest, time will turn things around and the value of the treatment and the wisdom of our decisions will emerge.

9

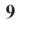

In 19 years of nursing I have never been so challenged and humbled by a group of patients as I have been by those who have epilepsy.

Almost all the patients I work with have medically refractory seizures. To see them courageously battling against their seizures is always inspiring to me. I have been deeply moved by their profound faith and strength. The possibility that patients may have a seizure when engaging in even the most basic daily activities cannot be dismissed. Things that we take for granted are dangerous for them and, at times, impossible. I often think about that when I drive my car, an activity prohibited for so many of my patients.

I have particularly admired those patients who manage to find humor in their seizures and who have invited me to share in their wit. And I am overjoyed when a patient achieves seizure control through medication or surgery, gains new energy, and makes progress in psychosocial areas.

One of my greatest lessons in dealing with epilepsy came from a woman who was a candidate for epilepsy surgery. Her diagnostic workup was delayed several times while we waited for some modifications to be made on the intracranial electrodes that would be used to localize her seizure onset. I apologized to her for the delay during a clinic visit and voiced my irritation over the whole matter. She looked at me calmly and said, "God's time is not our time. When He's ready, it'll happen." The electrodes eventually arrived, the patient's seizures were localized, and she had epilepsy surgery. Today, she is seizure-free and off anticonvulsants.

I often recall that woman's statement when I become impatient about deadlines or stressed because we are unsuccessful in controlling someone's seizures. My patient taught me to have faith and to be at peace with myself every day. And always to have hope.

10

Practicing in an American town close to Mexico, I find myself treating epilepsy of the borderlands. My fluency in Spanish keeps the waiting room full, even in these days of managed care. (Of course, it only takes two patients and their extended Mexican families to fill the waiting room!) The Spanish-speaking patients are often fearful when they come to the office because they expect another gringo doctor who can speak only five words of Spanish and yet thinks that he can effectively communicate. Once they realize that I speak fluent Spanish, out tumble all of the medical details that they couldn't push through the last doctor's translator. An explanation in clear Spanish calms them and the healing process begins, even before their new prescriptions are filled. For patients who have seizures, a doctor's explanations and willingness to discuss drug side effects cast light where only darkness lay before.

Seizures are caused by any lesion or scar that creates a short circuit in the brain. Hispanic seizure patients have the same range of disorders underlying their epilepsy as do other patients, but in the area where I live they are at particularly high risk for cysticercosis, a parasitic disease common in Latin America. In most people, cysticercosis causes a fairly harmless tapeworm infection. In some patients, however, the larvae escape the intestine to form cysts in muscles, the brain, and other organs. In the brain, the encysted larvae die fairly quickly, but in the process of dying they irritate the brain and cause seizures, stroke-like paralysis, or blockage of the cerebrospinal fluid, leading to hydrocephalus.

Mr. A was sent to me by his attorney. His seizures appeared to begin after he hit his head in a car accident. Each seizure started with shaking of both sides of his body followed by loss of consciousness. The sequence of his seizure behaviors prompted his previous physicians to dismiss his spells as fake. I was the third or fourth neurologist to see Mr. A but the first to actually talk with him, because he spoke only Spanish. Mr. A cared little about the legal case; he just wanted to return to his job as a draftsman for a blueprint company so that he could continue to support his family. An MRI showed a tiny cysticercosis cyst in the supplementary motor area, the one spot in the brain where a seizure can cause shaking on both sides of the body, without necessarily loss of consciousness. His seizures were real and responded well to seizure medicines.

Many of my patients purchase their medications across the border in Mexico, either to save money or because they see doctors in Mexico whose prescriptions must be filled there. Some seizure medications in Mexico are virtually identical to their counterparts in the United States, but other medicines have different names and strengths or are absorbed differently by the body. Most often these differences affect only dosing, but sometimes they can create problems.

I was once called to a certain hospital to see Mr. B, a Mexican who had been admitted from the ER the previous day after experiencing several recent seizures. The seizures had been controlled with a high dose of intravenous seizure medication, but I was asked to see him because a painful red rash now enveloped his entire body. In the ER record I noted that his family had informed the nurses that he was allergic to a Mexican seizure medicine. The emergency physician on duty didn't know that this was the *same* medicine (but known by a different name in Mexico) he had ordered be administered intravenously in the ER to Mr. B. I was angry because the patient went through needless suffering, but instead of screaming at the physician involved I sent a letter to the Chief of Staff (who was Mexican-American himself). Now their hospital policy requires checking with the pharmacy or Poison Control about any medicine, American or Mexican, that the ER staff doesn't recognize by name.

Most physicians across the border in Mexico are good clinicians. Patients who receive poor medical care suffer mostly from the lack of medical equipment, especially in the public hospitals. However, a few doctors are known for their poor judgment, even among their Mexican colleagues. Not long ago, I saw Miss C, a pretty young Mexican-

American who came to my office with her fiancé. She shyly told me about her spells of visual distortion, for which her family had insisted she see Dr. R, an older neurosurgeon in Mexico. Dr. R fancies himself a neurologist and he had obtained an EEG, told her that she had seizures, and immediately put her on a mixture of four different seizure medicines. The drug combination made her feel dizzy and, fortunately, she came back to the United States for a second opinion.

Reverently, the young woman's boyfriend offered me her EEG to review. The pages were splashed with electrical traces of coughs, swallows, and hiccups, but nothing that looked like seizure activity. Her visual symptoms appeared to suggest migraine headaches rather than seizures, so I took her off the seizure drugs (all four!) and put her on a migraine medicine. That cleared up her problems. The irony was that she lived in my city but had been sent to Mexico by her family because of Dr. R's "prestige" and because his fees were cheaper (slightly) than those of the American physicians. By the time the family paid for the unneeded EEG and four useless prescriptions, they had actually spent more than they would have if they had seen an American doctor in the first place.

Overall, my Spanish-speaking patients give me the most personal satisfaction. They are doubly grateful to me—for their medical care and for the interpersonal relationship that a common language permits. In turn, I find that they meet my latest drugs and medical gadgets with something enduring, ancient as the falling sickness itself. Here, the Latino population is as hardy and rooted as mesquite, their accommodation to place and disease as varied as the desert blooms. In a world where a slick, postindustrial sameness affects our movies, our malls, and our lives, my medical practice retains a special immediacy and flavor.

11

❖ ❖ ❖ ❖ ❖

My experiences with patients over the years have elicited emotions in me ranging from sadness to admiration.

At times, I have been overwhelmed by sadness. For example, a young patient in the prime of his life revealed to me that he felt God didn't like him and was punishing him with seizures. The young patient was lonely and had no friends. He was out of touch with people his own age and interacted only with his brother.

At times I feel very close to my patients. For example, once I saw a patient on a day that I did not usually schedule for office visits. I didn't know the woman very well. During the visit, which coincided with the anniversary of her father's death, the patient immediately opened up to me and revealed intimate details about her father's death. Her openness touched me, bringing tears to my eyes.

At other times, I admire the determination and courage that patients have shown. One such patient was a librarian. When she was having a seizure at work, she would remove some of her clothing. Yet despite this humiliating loss of self-control, she continued to return to work each day, never sure when this embarrassing episode would repeat itself.

I feel privileged when I realize that I play a prime role in the lives of many of my patients. As an indication of this closeness, I am often referred to by my first name. One time during a phone call, I could hear someone in the background say my first name. There was no confusion as to who I was. My last name wasn't necessary to identify me. It was as if I were a relative or close friend.

12

Laughing, my darling Linda twirls the jump rope for her nieces and nephews. Her father's roses unfold in the slanting sunlight, and the children frolic in the front yard grass.

Stepping back, Linda trips. She strikes her head on the bricks lining the flowerbed and then goes briefly out. The children run screaming for their grandparents in the house. Linda wakes up and seems fine except for a headache; she does not go to the hospital.

The staring spells begin a few months later. Linda's MRI scan does not show any abnormalities and her EEG is negative. My colleague tries to convince her that the spells are psychological, but I feel differently and start her on seizure medication. Her staring spells stop. Soon she trusts no other neurologist but me, her husband.

Later, the spells become drop attacks. Without warning, Linda drops limply to the floor and awakens confused. My son, Michael, watches as his stepmother goes down in the kitchen. Awakening, Linda does not recognize him or me. She regards us gravely but does not talk. Her confusion worries Michael more than her limp fall to the ground, but he watches me sit with her. He sits with her, too, and comforts her until she recognizes us and can speak. He learns to stay calm. Years later this will help him when his grandmother, alone with her grandchildren, has a massive heart attack—he will dial 911 himself, comfort her, and give a complete history to the paramedics when they arrive.

When seizures happen, we both feel helpless. The drop attacks come with no warning. Even a walk to the kitchen is dangerous. Seeing Linda's bruised face fills me with anger and guilt.

During the medical evaluation of Linda's drop attacks, a cardiologist rules out cardiac arrhythmia but reports her anyway to the Department of Motor Vehicles, in accordance with state law. I go to the Motor Vehicles hearing with Linda. As a physician, I have been sending patients to these hearings for years. I know that most of the hearings officers are reasonable people, but the impending bureaucratic ritual gnaws at our confidence. Maybe she'll get the one officer who just started last week or the one who hates doctors' wives. As it turns out, her hearing officer proves receptive to the logic of Linda's story and doesn't take away her driver's license. We can relax.

But not completely. Linda drives. She can stay up late but not too late; she can have one or two drinks but not more. Different seizure medications give her different side effects. One makes her tired, others make her dizzy and edgy. Every antibiotic, every late night, every big party has to be reviewed for its possible affect on her seizures.

How have these experiences changed my approach to doctoring? Even before Linda's spells, I cautiously considered the diagnosis of hysteria and believed that I was keenly aware of the importance of medication side effects and the significance of not being able to drive.

But the biggest impact of Linda's seizures on me as a physician has been to increase my awareness of the helplessness and anger that spouses and other family members feel about the illness itself. Now, when a patient's husband or wife comes screaming into the exam room wanting to know why someone didn't fix his or her spouse's seizures (or headaches or back pain or brain tumor) *yesterday*, I can choke down my own rising anger and empathize with the enraged person. Nine times out of ten we can succeed in forging an effective partnership to fight the real enemy—the crackling, uncontrolled electricity in the brain that underlies seizures.

As a family member, I am still learning the same lessons over and over again: We are fragile beings made of seawater clinging to a skeleton of chalk. Tidal rhythms still tug us at the cellular level, and no more than a heartbeat separates us from the morgue. Each day we live is a treasure, and each day lived with the people we love is a treasure beyond price.

13

I am a pediatric neurologist and treat a wide variety of neurologic disorders in children, including epilepsy. I feel close to all my patients but especially to my patients with epilepsy and to their parents. In part this is because of the nature of epilepsy and its treatment (recurrent seizures necessitating telephone calls, frequent visits to the office to adjust medications, and so on), and in part this is because I share in the hopes, achievements, and frustrations of my patients and their parents. I come to know many of them intimately.

Rather than dread the initial consultation with parents whose child has just had his or her first seizure, I welcome the opportunity. I try to explain what the disorder is, how it comes about, how it is treated, and how, together, we can face the challenges ahead. Almost immediately, I try to defuse the word *epilepsy* by explaining that it is a Greek word for seizures and that although it carries a special mystique or stigma, it means nothing more than recurring seizures. I believe it is better for the family (and later the child) to have heard the term epilepsy right from the beginning rather than to have it whispered to them or thrust on them by a well-meaning teacher or acquaintance.

When I am discussing the nature of seizures with my young patients, I try to use age-appropriate analogies to help explain how a "short circuit" can cause a seizure and how the brain is left unchanged after the event. Over the years I have used the analogy of radio static but I find that kids now have little knowledge of radios, much less static. Or, I liken a seizure to "snow" or "interference" on a television screen (also a passé analogy in the age of transistors) as a graphic way of explaining a temporary electric discharge that activates the brain in an unwanted manner. Certain comic books (for example, Seizure Man and Dottie the Dalmatian) have been immensely beneficial as educational tools for younger children, and I am grateful to the Epilepsy Foundation of America for these and other informative brochures that help kids and their parents as they attempt to cope with the diagnosis of epilepsy.

I have had my share of triumphs in caring for children with epilepsy. In some situations I believe my knowledge and judgment changed the outcome significantly, and I take special pride in sharing the joy of a patient whose life has done a complete turnaround.

I think of Bobby, who came to me after suffering several generalized tonic–clonic seizures. He bravely battled on, refusing to give up his usual activities despite several seizures a month. He participated in a tennis tournament and in a hockey match in Canada. His mother left her job and wore a beeper so that she could respond to the frantic calls from Bobbie's school when he experienced another seizure. But she never let him know how desperate she felt about what was happening to him.

Bobby experienced many more seizures before I realized that his EEG, which had been considered by his previous neurologists to be consistent with partial epilepsy, actually showed generalized rather than focal epileptiform abnormalities. This suggested to me that his seizures would likely respond to an altogether different drug from the ones he had been taking before. After I changed Bobby's medicine, his seizures stopped for good. It is now 6 years later and Bobby takes no medications. He's a sophomore at a prestigious Ivy League college, studying to be a physician, of course!

I also think of situations in which I have failed to help children who have countless seizures and who show some regression in their cognitive development. Ironically, the doctor–patient bond is strongest with these children and their parents. I try to give them, as my mentor taught me, a bit of myself whenever the latest anti-convulsant fails and when the learning and behavioral difficulties escalate.

This branch of medicine is not without its tragedies, too. I have vivid memories of attending the wake for Robert, whose seizures appeared to be improving little by little but who was found dead one morning, probably having succumbed to cardiac arrest in the midst of a seizure. I remember Diane, who drowned in her bathtub, probably also during a seizure, just as her mother left the room to answer the telephone. At such times I search my conscience and ask whether I did enough; whether a different medical regimen, per-haps in the hands of a different physician, would have spared this child's life.

But there are also the light moments. I will never forget seeing a 10-year-old boy, the nephew of a colleague, who had possible ab-sence seizures. These seizures had been noted by his teacher but, cu-riously, not by his family. During the office visit, I asked him to hy-perventilate (a common technique for bringing on an absence seizure) and within a minute he had a full-fledged absence seizure, lasting almost 30 seconds. It was so dramatic to me that I couldn't help asking his mother, who had observed the seizure with me, why she had never noticed these spells. "Oh, of course I saw them, doc-tor. But since everyone in our family meditates, I just thought Joshua was meditating, too!"

Being a doctor for children with epilepsy is a special privilege. It enables me to involve myself in many facets of each patient's life, helping the child to negotiate the obstacles at every stage of devel-opment that the disorder sometimes brings. It also enables me to help the family as they learn to encourage the child's growth, development, and eventual autonomy, and as they advocate for their child at school and in the community.

It is a rare privilege indeed, and one for which I have been most grateful.

14

Epilepsy affects millions of people in a wide variety of ways. Some people experience minimal change in their lives but others suffer monumental upheavals. We can expect that, when a child receives a diagnosis of epilepsy, the parents and siblings of the child will also be affected. The literature describes many of these expected changes and provides specific strategies for health-care professionals to use in helping the family to adjust to the inevitable changes that occur after the diagnosis.

Our literature is much less useful, however, in helping us to understand what happens to a family when children with epilepsy become adults and yet continue to be dependent on their parents. Sometimes this relationship between parent and adult child is a continuation of an unhealthy set of behaviors established early in the patient's childhood. For others, this extended relationship is both healthy and essential. Whatever the outcome, the truth is that we are not expert at dealing with the needs of these newly defined families. Four examples come to mind.

Mrs. R is 65 years old, and Linda, her 42-year-old daughter, has a lifelong history of complex partial seizures. Linda has three children and lives with her mother and her father, who is also disabled. Mrs. R is now the breadwinner and caretaker for this three-generation household. She works part-time, draws on government support for the remainder of her needs, and provides the main support for the family.

Mrs. K is 60 years old and cares for her adult, moderately retarded daughter, who as a child was given the diagnosis of Lennox–Gastaut syndrome. The daughter continues to have seizures and is confined to a wheelchair. During our first interview I acquired all the usual medical information about Mrs. K's daughter. Then I asked Mrs. K about herself—her health, her feelings, and what backup plans she had for her daughter's care in the event that she had even a minor illness. She looked at me with tears in her eyes as she said, "No one has ever asked me anything like that before."

Mrs. J is 45 years old and has two sons with epilepsy. She brings them to the clinic one at a time because she finds that managing both of them together is too difficult. Neither child is seizure-free, and both are mildly to moderately retarded. Mrs. J is a widow; her husband was murdered when the boys were toddlers. Her main support is from members of her church.

Finally, I think of Mr. A, a 65-year-old retired seaman. His 25-year-old son, Kevin who is moderately retarded and has intractable seizures, lives with him. Kevin's mother died 20 years earlier. Mr. A continues to provide constant support for his son.

What I find most striking is how these parents have been called on to cope with their chronically ill children for such an extended period. Certainly, parents expect to carry most of the burden of caring for their child when the child is young. What they don't expect, however, is that their responsibilities will continue at the same level of intensity throughout their child's life. As these parents grow older their own developmental tasks are placed on hold because they are trapped in a constant state of child rearing. Their personal needs to grow and move on are frequently unmet, and developmental conflicts are left unresolved.

My respect for these parents grows with every visit. My fears for them also increase. They have devoted themselves to the care of their children and continue, for more than 40 years in some cases, to bear the burden. I have been impressed by their selfless devotion under circumstances that are more difficult than many others could tolerate.

What have I learned from working with these parents? On a personal level, I am constantly grateful to them for showing me the strength of their human spirit. Their love, creativity, and ability to solve seemingly insurmountable problems are inspirational. More important, working with these families has helped me to focus my care not only on the family as a unit but on each member of the family individually. My practice responsibilities are meant to help the person with epilepsy. However, in these cases I also now profile the parents. I get to know them well enough to understand their feelings, fears, and concerns. Because they tend to be somewhat neglectful of their own health, we take time to discuss healthy behaviors. I encourage them to obtain regular checkups.

By working with parents, I indirectly influence the care of their adult child and potentially improve everyone's overall situation. When we provide additional, needed support and help for these devoted parents, we also help the patient more.

15

As a nurse with no previous experience with neurology patients, I was very uneasy at the prospect of caring for patients with epilepsy. Yet here I was, about to assume responsibility for a patient with active seizures, getting a report on the patient from the nurse going off duty and finding myself becoming increasingly anxious as the nature of my patient's seizures was described to me. I was anxious about the unpredictable nature of seizures, not about what I needed to do for the patient in the event of a seizure. No matter how closely I watched the patient, he or she could suddenly and unexpectedly have a seizure and perhaps be badly injured.

I found that the best way to overcome my anxiety was to spend as much time as possible with my patient, getting to know him or her as a person, rather than gathering all the information I could about epilepsy in general. Doing that replaced my tension and anxiety with respect for my patient and how he or she lived. Then, when my patient had a seizure, I felt that I was taking care of the *person*, not the seizure.

I often find myself thinking about the general public and how little they know about epilepsy. I'm sure they equate epilepsy with grand mal seizures. I wonder if a bystander would respond with compassion and come to the aid of the victim if the bystander were to witness a grand mal event. I also question how someone would react to witnessing one of the other types of seizures that we see in the hospital. How would my patient be treated if he or she acted out in public in the midst of a seizure? Would this person be treated in the same compassionate manner as here in the controlled environment of the hospital? How would I react? I *hope* that I would react appropriately in that situation.

I can't help admiring these patients and their families for living with a disability that touches every aspect of their lives.

16

My patients have taught me a great deal about how people who are disadvantaged live in our society. Many of my patients are indigent and have problems obtaining sufficient food and adequate housing; troubles with drugs, crime, and familial discord can affect their attitudes toward their seizures. Contrary to what their doctors may think, seizures may not be the most important threat in their lives and taking seizure medications properly and establishing good daily habits may therefore not rank high on their list of priorities.

The physician who recognizes this fact will avoid the frustration of trying to help patients who do not *seem* to want to help themselves. This point becomes even more important when patients appear to engage in self-destructive behavior. The "shoot-yourself-in-the-foot" phenomenon is apparent in some patients whose lives have been so troubled that they do not feel comfortable when medical treatment is successful and, therefore, they seek out further trouble. One of my patients, Jose, was forever noncompliant because he felt it was not macho to take medicine. After a decade I finally convinced him to change that attitude and he became compliant. Then he developed a new problem—the uncomfortable feeling of success. His successful treatment gave way to renewed noncompliance, not because of macho feelings but seemingly to seek out more trouble.

All of us become used to our living conditions, even if they represent the ultimate in chaos and difficulty. Accommodating to these conditions psychologically leads patients to become noncompliant and unable to handle any kind of success. This phenomenon can be a real challenge for the epileptologist.

Indeed, these unfortunate attitudes can be understood in terms of the most inclusive and important rule of human behavior: people treat the outside world the same way they think the outside world has treated them. Furthermore, people may also treat *themselves* the way they think the outside world has treated them. Thus, trouble from the outside world brings on self-destructive behavior, often exacerbated by the patient's negative actions toward others.

The role of the epileptologist is to break this negative cycle. Then, when patients experience a few triumphs (it is hoped) in the treatment of their seizures and acquire insight into their self-destructive behavior, they will seek out further success.

17

❖ ❖ ❖ ❖ ❖

I first met Billy when he showed up with his mother in the outpatient neurology clinic. Billy couldn't sit still. He bounced off the walls, jumped up and down on the examination bed and the floor, and picked at the ophthalmoscope (and any other object within reach). He came over to my table and played with the pens and pads of paper. He just wouldn't stay in one place. His mother looked well weathered beyond her years. She must have been in her late thirties but had the deep, tired lines in her face of someone years older. She spent the first visit filling me in on the history of Billy's epilepsy, all the while telling Billy to sit still.

Billy was 8 years old. He had frequent staring spells at home and at school that could be brought on by photic stimulation and the least bit of hyperventilation. Although I started him on a seizure medication before long he had the first of many tonic–clonic seizures. I switched him to a different medication and saw him frequently in the office to monitor his medication and seizures.

Billy's staring spells decreased but he was not doing well in school because he couldn't pay attention in class and was easily distracted. I told Billy that he should sit at the front of the class, which he did. There, at least, his attention was more prolonged.

Then Billy's epilepsy worsened. He began to have more frequent tonic–clonic seizures and was doing even less well in school. He eventually enrolled in another school that was better adapted to his needs.

As he entered adolescence, Billy had a growth spurt and changed from a small, hyperactive, tousled-haired boy to a tall, gangly adolescent with acne and an increasing interest in clothes and girls. But he also had intractable tonic–clonic seizures and marked attention deficit. He rebelled against his mother, refused to take his medicines, and acted out in school.

Back then when I met with Billy, his mother, and his younger, cute-as-a-button sister (who also bounced off the office walls during appointments), his voice would break, changing back and forth between his previous soprano and his new tenor. He was barely keeping up in school. He never complained that his classmates were treating him any differently because of his seizures, but he had made only a few friends. His mother sought me out, justifiably, at the clinic or by telephone several times a month. Once she brought her other daughter with her, who was older than Billy and a spitting image of herself except that she was black. This elder daughter also had tonic–clonic seizures and a winsome smile but moved to Virginia to live with her father.

Meanwhile, the nurses at Billy's special school noted that he was having more frequent tonic–clonic seizures. Increasing the dosage of his seizure medication to achieve high, even supratherapeutic, serum levels did not suppress his seizures. On one occasion, Billy was taken to the hospital in status epilepticus. Another time he was admitted with toxic encephalopathy, triphasic waves on his EEG, and normal serum ammonia but a high level of his seizure drug.

Over time, the background rhythms on Billy's EEGs began to slow. I had a nagging suspicion that he might have an underlying metabolic or genetic disorder in addition to his epilepsy. Sadly, though, before I could admit Billy to the hospital again for further evaluation, I was called at 6 o'clock one morning by the morgue. Billy had been found dead by his mother, face down and blue. Before his body could be moved to the funeral home, I had to certify the cause of his death. I was asked to do this over the phone. Somewhat taken aback and not used to certifying death without seeing the patient, I said that I would be there shortly.

I drove to the desolate part of town where Billy's family lived. There, in front of the undertakers, was an inconsolable mother, a tearful elder daughter, and Billy's little sister, who was running around examining everything, clearly not aware of what had happened. I reached out to touch Billy's mother, who threw her arms around me and sobbed.

The undertaker took me aside and we went down to the cold room where Billy lay stiff and quiet. Being primarily an adult neurologist, I was used to elderly and terminal patients meeting what was usually a not unexpected death. Here, outside the hospital setting, in an undertaker's cold room, seeing a young man whom I had followed almost monthly for the last 7 to 8 years, I found it difficult to believe that Billy was suddenly gone, his young face a mixture of blue mottling and adolescent acne. He was still the gangly adolescent whom I remembered.

The next day, a simple ceremony was held in the chapel above the morgue. Fifty or sixty people, mostly members of Billy's church, sat in fold-up chairs, numb. The gathering included a mix of people that I wasn't used to seeing in this city. Half were black, half were white, and all were there because of their bond to the church and its social activities. Billy lay in his best Sunday clothes at the front. His mother and elder sister stood in front, shaking everyone's hands and wiping the tears from their faces. Someone was taking care of the little sister, who was running to and fro.

The pastor praised Billy in a somewhat abstract but warm fashion. Then, one of Billy's teachers from the church stood up. He was a young, energetic black man who talked eloquently and simply about those special qualities that Billy had that many in the audience, including me, didn't know about. Billy had been a dedicated participant in his church group and was studying to join the church. His teacher described the questions that Billy had discussed with him in private about the meaning of life and God. The room was silent.

At the end of the ceremony, Billy's mother came over again and introduced me to the closest and most important people in her life. I was Billy's doctor, she said. Surprisingly, I felt somewhat embarrassed. I suppose that I had wanted to come to pay my own respects to Billy and now, being identified as his doctor, I felt that somehow I was responsible for his death or at least that I had failed him. But many seemed touched and almost grateful that someone else from beyond their community—someone from the establishment—was there.

It was a peaceful but most unhappy day. I walked out into the thin, weak sunlight of early spring. There was no growth on the trees or on the ground. I walked out of the building and left Billy behind, forever dressed in his finest Sunday clothes.

I saw Billy's mother a couple more times. She came to the clinic just to see me and to hug me. Clinic had always been an important part of her social life, but now the link was broken. I told her to stop by for a chat anytime, if she wanted, but I suspected that, as time went on and her life moved on, our bond would weaken.

And so it has. The cement remained, but the bricks were gone.

18

I am a social worker, and even after 20 years of working with people who have epilepsy I still cannot escape the anxiety and apprehension that I feel each time I sit across from a patient in my office with the door closed. My patients and I seek a trusting, close interaction as we talk about illness, fears, and hopes. But when the door to my office closes, I never know whether we will achieve this desired intimacy or if the person will have a seizure.

When a seizure occurs, there are no familiar anchors for me. We are forced to abandon the usual rules of politeness, control, and predictability that I dearly value in my own personal life. I am left feeling helpless because even my best efforts can't halt the event. My anxiety is palpable as I worry that the patient might need the kind of medical attention that goes beyond my training.

Even more significantly under those circumstances, I feel uncomfortably voyeuristic. I find myself shifting my perspective: The person before me is transformed from a socially intact person into a patient within the sterile hospital environment. For what may last moments or minutes, I am compelled to watch this person, who is suddenly stripped of his or her usual social and physical veneers, in the grip of abnormal electrical activity that, like a powerful magnet, takes control. I want to avert my eyes, as if doing so would spare the person some loss of dignity. I was not invited to witness this most private moment, yet I am part of that moment and leaving is not an option for me. My only emotional escape is to observe the patient from a clinical distance.

When the seizure ends, I awkwardly attempt to reset our interaction and to return our relationship to where it had been before the seizure. However, even my best efforts fall short because there is an inescapable residue left behind. The playing field is now tilted. I must draw on my training to level the field again, so that feelings and experiences can be put into meaningful words.

If our work is to be successful, I must create an atmosphere in which even the unspeakable can be uttered and explored. The patient knows, as do I, that witnessing the seizure has added another layer to our relationship. In our ongoing work together, we both must accept the risks inherent in each encounter if we are to achieve the insights that transcend the seizure.

19

My work with patients with epilepsy is challenging, intellectually stimulating, and thoroughly enjoyable. What distinguishes epilepsy from most other chronic illnesses? Epilepsy is essentially about losing control.

As humans, we struggle to achieve control over ourselves and our environment. Unfortunately, the nature of epilepsy is that periodically, and at random intervals, patients lose this struggle by surrendering control of their bodies and their minds. Because seizures can happen anywhere and at any time, for some people epilepsy becomes the focal point of their lives. And, like patients with other chronic illnesses, patients with epilepsy wonder what they could have done to bring this condition on themselves or their families.

This is one reason why I try to encourage my patients to regain as much control over their epilepsy as possible. From the first moment I meet a patient, I stress that my role is to help him or her understand what is going on by educating the patient as much as possible. I explain that when the patient is comfortable with this knowledge, he or she will make some of the treatment decisions. My patients have told me that they are frightened at first to be in charge of their own care but then come to cherish the feeling of control engendered by being in charge.

I inform my patients that the majority of persons with epilepsy lead normal, happy, and productive lives. This is a difficult point to make because most people with epilepsy who do well choose not to disclose the fact that they have epilepsy to many other people. I think that the lack of visible role models makes it more difficult for patients whose seizures aren't well controlled and for young people with well-controlled epilepsy to be accepted into society.

I am part of a group of health-care providers who devote most of their time to epilepsy. This dedicated group includes physicians, research and clinical nurses, social workers, neuropsychologists, psychiatrists, and resource specialists. Being part of this group contributes to the satisfaction that I feel in working with adults and children with epilepsy. We, in turn, are privileged to work in a hospital that allows us to be generous with the time and services that we can provide to our patients. I have never had to turn away a patient because the person had no money. And I have never had to say, "I'd like to be able to provide this for you, but we don't have it available here."

The most difficult thing that I have to deal with is ignorance on the part of people who should know better. Because of this ignorance, persons with epilepsy are discriminated against in many ways. It is understandable that many members of the public have major mis-conceptions about epilepsy. What I find amazing, though, is that many of my nonepileptologist colleagues—people with medical knowledge and training—also have tremendous misconceptions about epilepsy. Many of my patients have come into our emergency room (an emergency room belonging to a major teaching affiliate of one of the world's best-known medical institutions) only to have their acute medical problems attributed entirely to epilepsy—prob-lems such as heart attacks and strokes. Yet they would have been at-tended to in minutes had they not carried the diagnosis of epilepsy.

One of the most outrageous examples I've seen of discrimination against someone with epilepsy occurred when one of my older and otherwise healthy patients unexpectedly died at home. This death was not investigated by the medical examiner because, he reasoned, people with epilepsy "sometimes die suddenly." Another patient of mine with epilepsy died at home one evening. He was an otherwise healthy young man. This death also was not investigated. Because the young man had epilepsy it was called a natural death. To allow the unexpected deaths of otherwise healthy people in the community pass without performing a thorough investigation seems criminal to me. How many of them are dying unnecessarily?

Discrimination based on sex, race, or physical handicap is no longer considered acceptable. However, people with epilepsy face discrimination every day. I work with many children and adults who face these obstacles and yet manage to live happy lives. Others aren't so fortunate, however.

I'm starting to realize how underappreciated quality-of-life issues are in the care of patients with epilepsy. For some patients a single seizure is unacceptable, whereas for others the side effects that they must accept to achieve a seizure-free life are intolerable. Whatever the expectation of my patient, the joy that I feel when he or she comes into the office seizure-free for the first time is impossible to put into words.

There is another gratifying aspect to caring for patients with epilepsy. They are immensely grateful. They are grateful for being treated fairly and with honesty and respect. My co-workers, who have been at this longer than I have, taught me this by example. My patients are amazingly selfless and willing to do anything, not just because they feel that it will help them but because they feel that it may help others. Their sense of altruism is ever present.

I have had some patients for whom a seizure-free life is still an unattainable goal despite our best efforts. I expect such people to be disappointed not only in their condition but also in me. I sometimes wonder if they will blame me because I have not been able to treat their seizures successfully. But I am always surprised. These patients are often the *most* grateful: grateful for the other services that we can provide; grateful to have a place where they can go; grateful that no matter what, we will always be there for them. They have often lived a long time with their epilepsy and have learned to cope with their lot in life. They amaze me with their gratitude for my continued efforts to try to help them.

Helping patients can take many different forms. I have one patient who walked into the office for her first appointment and told me that she had "pseudoseizures." In the course of monitoring her seizures, we took her off seizure medication and waited a few days. She went on to have several of her typical seizures, which clearly appeared to be partial-onset seizures on the EEG. With proper anticonvulsant treatment over the next year, she made tremendous progress with her life. Just knowing that her events were epileptic and not psychiatric in origin was helpful to her.

By contrast, I have another patient whose epilepsy had been treated for many years with several anticonvulsants. She had experienced a variety of side effects from these medicines. Her medical history suggested that her seizures were not stereotypical. I admitted her to the hospital, tapered her off anticonvulsants, and observed her during video/EEG monitoring. It was quite evident that her events were provoked by interactions with certain members of her family. I sat down with her and discussed the idea that stress can cause behaviors that look to others like seizures. She was most receptive to this idea. After she was discharged from the hospital, she was able to accept that her events were stress-related behaviors rather than seizures. She has made tremendous progress. Correcting the misdiagnosis of epilepsy was as important for her as making the appropriate diagnosis of epilepsy was to the first patient.

When I find myself dealing with a patient whom I find particularly difficult, I spend a little time trying to imagine myself in that person's situation. Doing this often relieves much of the tension or stress I feel and has taught me that people who live with epilepsy—patients, their families, and friends—deserve our utmost respect and admiration.

People with chronic illness can be difficult to deal with and may sometimes choose not to do what we recommend. But it is they who must live with the consequences of deciding whether or not to become active partners in their treatment. They, more than I, should have the right to make decisions about what they do and do not want to do. I have had patients tell me that they were frightened to come back for followup because they thought that I was going to be angry at something they did on their own, such as changing or stopping their medication. I explain that I don't get angry about these things because I'm not the one who has to live with the consequences of their actions—they are. I emphasize that I make recommendations to them, not demands. I find that this approach helps my own mental well-being as well as my relationship with patients, and I hope that this approach helps them feel free to tell me whatever is going on or is on their minds. They know that I appreciate how side effects that others might find trivial may significantly impair their ability to lead a happy and functional life.

Working with people with epilepsy has immensely rewarded me. I have gained as much from my patients as I hope they have gained from me. I look forward to seeing my patients. Although I am also interested in epilepsy research, my life would not be complete without working directly with patients. I only hope that I can teach them as much as I have learned from them.

20

❖ ❖ ❖ ❖ ❖

I started working with epilepsy patients about a year ago and have found that although they each have individual personalities, they all fear their next seizure, wondering when and if it will occur and if the medication they're taking is really going to work.

I have also found that health-care professionals forget that some patients with epilepsy cannot do basic things that the rest of us take for granted. Imagine not being able to drive or not being allowed to hold your child or grandchild in your arms because you might drop the child. I sympathize with and try to empathize with my patients. I think to myself, "How would I feel in that situation?" I know that I wouldn't like the feeling of losing control.

I feel a special bond with particular patients. When they first come into the office, they are frightened or tired from a recent seizure or from the medication that they're taking. As I come to know them and help them with challenges in their lives, I gain a new perspective on my own life. As a result, I have learned to be grateful for my blessings. I reflect on how fortunate I am because I don't have to fear seizures, I don't have certain privileges or rights taken away from me, and I don't have to be concerned about injuring myself. Having such fears must be very scary.

I've learned a lot from these patients. I have also learned quite a bit about the disorder itself and how the public views it. I find it all very fascinating and interesting. Patients with epilepsy persevere in the face of their illness. Many of them are very motivated to combat their epilepsy in any way possible. And when my patients' seizures become controlled, I share their joy and excitement and feel that I'm part of their life.

Remarkably, some patients with uncontrolled seizures can still smile, have a good attitude and a sense of humor, and inspire the people that surround them and care for them. People like me.

21

In our epilepsy clinic, certain occasions create an atmosphere of happy excitement. One of these is when a patient brings in his or her school class picture, which is then added to our gallery. Another cause for celebration is a patient passing the 1-year anniversary of being seizure-free, a requirement in our state before someone with seizures can legally drive. Whenever my staff informs me of these events or of engagements, weddings, or births in the families of our seizure patients, it reminds me that these events are more important to the patients than taking medication or keeping diaries of their clinical attacks.

Of all such special office visits, I most enjoy those from patients who have just graduated. For at least one moment, I can share in the student's (and the family's) accomplishment, such as the successful completion of another school year, graduation from college, or completion of postgraduate studies despite a daily struggle against epilepsy.

These occasions are bittersweet, however, when I recall one young patient who never made it to graduation. She chose to disregard my medical counseling and the pleading of her fiancé and parents about observing her medication regimen, getting adequate rest, eating regular meals, and avoiding potentially life-threatening situations. One evening she neglected to take her medications and went swimming alone. She had a seizure and drowned. She was barely 20 years old.

But then I remember another young woman who, as a child of 11, was brought to the emergency room in absence status epilepticus. Fortunately she responded well to medication. The patient and her parents faithfully followed my instructions about her medication, office visits, and lab work. The girl remained seizure-free through middle school, high school, and college.

When I think of her and of other young students who have assumed personal responsibility for controlling their seizures, I wish I knew where they were today so that I could thank them for their courage, persistence, and compliance.

22

Decades ago, physicians began to recognize the connection between abnormal brain function and diseases of other organ systems, such as the heart, lungs, or liver. This connection helped to explain why, for example, patients with chronic renal failure experienced headache, lethargy, and occasionally coma.

At that time, hemodialysis was introduced as an experimental treatment for end-stage renal disease. I was training to be an EEG technician and became involved in a study of dialysis patients to determine whether EEG changes correlated with the neurologic improvement associated with successful dialysis treatment.

The first patient to volunteer for the study was Mr. Pappas, a young Greek businessman with no previous history of neurologic disease. He underwent hemodialysis over a period of 4 months. My task was to perform an EEG every other day. Although he was extremely sick, Mr. Pappas remained stoic during the procedure, tolerating the measurement of his head, the acetone, the collodion, the abrasion of his scalp, and my clumsiness as a student.

Mr. Pappas spoke English moderately well but still felt uncomfortable with his limited vocabulary and accent. I began to help him with English and he, in turn, taught me some Greek phrases. No matter how exhausted he was, he always put forth extra effort to improve his English. In fact, the only error he ever made was to call me "Eddie," which was the name of one of my fellow students. Even after I made two or three attempts to politely correct him, he persisted. Therefore, to Mr. Pappas and his family, I became Eddie. I accepted that nickname as their personal gift and was even more moved when one day he said to a Greek hospital attendant, "Eddie ine kalo pedi" (Eddie's a good boy).

Early one morning, a nursing student entered Mr. Pappas' room while it was still dark. She flipped on the light switch and the fluorescent bulb above his head flickered. For the first time, the muscles of his face, limbs, and trunk began to jerk violently. Within 1 or 2 days his kidney function worsened and the myoclonic jerks evolved to major, generalized seizures. Fortunately, the major seizures stopped when the dialysis treatment was adjusted.

Up until then, Mr. Pappas' resting EEGs had never shown any epileptiform activity. He became too sensitive to standard photic stimulation to safely incorporate it into an EEG study. Nevertheless, he indicated that he knew how important that part of the procedure was for the test and courageously volunteered to continue with stro-

boscopic stimulation. He and I agreed that I would perform a modi-
fied technique of waving a low-intensity flashlight once or twice
across his closed eyes. This technique turned out to be enough to
evoke abnormalities without inducing full seizures. Indeed, this
technique was used successfully to monitor changes in brain ex-
citability during his hemodialysis and was adopted for all subsequent
patients in that research project.

Tragically, Mr. Pappas suffered further complications of his renal
disease, eventually became comatose, and died at the age of 38. Just
after he died, his wife, still shaking, stepped into the corridor and
stopped me from entering his room to pay my respects, saying, "You
good boy, Eddie, but you no come see Mr. Pappas no more. Mr. Pappas, he no more."

Four years later, an 11-year-old boy was referred to the EEG laboratory for assessment of inattentiveness at school. His previous
grades had been above average but he had begun to fail most sub-
jects. His handwriting had deteriorated to an uninterpretable mixture
of letters and scrawls. Although teachers suspected that he was
chronically depressed over the death of a family member several
years earlier, the psychiatrist thought his problems were due to a
neurologic disorder.

The boy was sent for a standard EEG, but it was obvious that the
request was for a test that could prove whether there was a relationship between his poor attention and handwriting and any brain wave
irregularities. When the boy was brought to the lab by the hospital
volunteer, I explained the procedure to him and applied the scalp
electrodes through his thick black hair. One aspect of this test was
different from a standard EEG: Instead of having him lie supine on
the hospital bed, I asked him to sit on the swivel chair in front of the
EEG machine.

I dictated some words for the boy to write with a red felt marking
pen near the lower channels of the moving EEG paper (while his
brain activity was being recorded). Soon, the mechanical sounds associated with normal EEG patterns were suddenly replaced for a few
seconds by the unmistakable clicking and scratching of the EEG
pens as they drew high-amplitude, classic three-per-second spike
and wave activity. During this absence seizure he stopped writing on
the EEG paper but quickly resumed his task after the normal EEG

rhythms reappeared. I felt personal satisfaction in knowing that the interpreting physician would have enough information to notify this child's teachers that the cause of his inattentiveness was not emotional but rather absence seizures.

While I removed the electrodes, the hospital volunteer arrived to pick up the EEG tracing for the medical director of the seizure clinic. A few minutes later I walked the boy back to the medical director's office. He had already analyzed the results and had begun to explain to the boy's mother that the test I performed had determined why her child was performing poorly in school.

It was only when I looked closely at her tired smile, still framed in a black veil, that I recognized her. She gave me the familiar look of approval for my technical contribution to her son's care. It also appeared that she remembered my efforts on behalf of her husband, Mr. Pappas, a few years before.

Before she left the clinic, clutching the new prescription for the medication that would stop her son's seizures, she simply said, "Thanks again, Eddie. You still a good boy."

23

I have cared for several patients who led productive, satisfying lives despite having several seizures a day. It has been particularly rewarding to follow some of these patients as they proceeded through the evaluation for epilepsy surgery and then became seizure-free after surgery, because they were then able to expand their horizons even further.

For example, one of my patients had experienced complex partial seizures since childhood. She had daily episodes of staring, along with automatisms, confused behavior, and amnesia. Once or twice a month her seizures secondarily generalized. After she had experienced a seizure while alone, panic symptoms developed that typically occurred when she was alone in her parking garage or in other isolated places. Despite her symptoms, she continued to work full time to support her family and raise several children. After epilepsy surgery she became seizure-free. When she saw me back in the office, she remarked on her new-found freedoms, including being able to travel alone to the Midwest (from Washington, DC) to accept an award from her corporation for outstanding work performance. She lives each day free from the fears that pervaded her life before surgery.

Then there are stories that are not as upbeat but equally memorable. One of my patients underwent a left temporal lobectomy with intraoperative language mapping. Although her surgery and mapping were uneventful, the day after her operation she became acutely withdrawn and extremely dysnomic. She was able to partially comprehend what was said to her but could not respond coherently. A brain MRI scan showed no acute changes but the serum level of her seizure medication was quite high, offering a possible explanation for her unusual behavior. When I went to find her in the MRI suite, I couldn't locate her. Unattended for a moment, she had left her stretcher. Along with my neurosurgical colleague and the radiology technologists, I frantically searched the entire neuroradiology area and eventually found her locked inside a changing room. I coaxed her into unlocking the door and found her sitting in a ball in a corner of the room. She was frightened and inconsolable.

Several days later, both her mood and language had improved and she related to me the frustration that she felt at not being able to communicate, as well as her fear that her language deficits would be permanent. I shared her frustrations. As her physician, I had felt perplexed (as to her condition), responsible (for not previously communicating to her all the possible negative outcomes of surgery), and quite helpless.

24

❖ ❖ ❖ ❖ ❖

Although the epilepsy protocol has been completed for my patient and my role as his study nurse is winding down, I still find myself gravitating to the same chair in front of the video monitor that gave me a full view of him during the study. Only now, when I glance up, the screen is blank and I don't have to worry. At least not until the next patient begins the study.

Over a year ago, when I first began to take care of persons with epilepsy, I was frightened about what I might see. When a patient moved a certain way while on camera, I was immediately at the bed-side. Many times a smiling person who was merely turning in bed greeted me. Other times I needed to react quickly because the patient was seizing.

I had been a nurse for almost 10 years but had had no experience with epilepsy before becoming involved with patients enrolled in a drug study for medically refractory seizures. Fortunately, many wonderful patients taught me about their disorder during the course of the study. I never realized how many different ways a seizure could manifest itself. Sometimes a patient would stop our conversa-tion and matter-of-factly state that a seizure had just occurred. What seizure? *I* didn't see anything.

The first generalized seizure that I witnessed seemed to last for-ever, although the clock registered only a little over a minute. I came away drained from the event. I cannot even imagine what it must feel like to experience such a seizure.

After watching my patient have this seizure, I had an overwhelm-ing need to protect him and my other patients from future harm. I was so afraid that patients would be injured while having a seizure that I tended to limit their activity too much. Luckily, the patients un-der my care understood my need to be protective. Looking back, I re-alize that the restrictions I placed on my patients would not have been ones that *I* could have accepted. Imagine someone talking to you through the door as you tried to take a shower; someone trying to escort you every time you took a walk in the hallway; or someone reminding you to move back into camera range. Yet that is exactly what I did to my patients!

But because I monitored my patients so closely I was able to de-velop a trusting relationship with them. Many patients were very open with me about their epilepsy and how it had affected their lives. Some patients inspired me with their stories, whereas others left me sad. Often I learned a great deal just by watching a family member guide a loved one through a seizure.

It's been a year since the study ended. I still think about the patients whom I took care of and wonder how they are doing on the new drugs. Have they returned to work? Are some of them driving?

Although the camera monitor is off, I can still see my patients in my mind and thank them for the knowledge, skills, and insights that they gave me and that will remain with me always.

25

At one time or another, working with patients and families affected by epilepsy evokes all the emotions known to humankind. And I'm sure that patients and their families (or caretakers) also experience each of these emotions as well.

I am thrilled when I see my patient's life turn around after an adjustment is made in his or her medication. And I am ecstatic when seizure surgery is successful in granting my patient total independence or a significant improvement in quality of life.

And then I am profoundly saddened when seizures take their toll, either by causing sudden unexplained death or severe injury. Both of these situations also make me feel helpless, even though I know I tried everything possible.

I feel frustrated when a patient's seizures don't come under control as much as I'd like, or when there is no drug study that is just right for a particular patient, or when surgery is not an option, or when surgery was tried but failed.

Another emotion I feel is one that patients and their caretakers often have: anger. They feel angry because they have epilepsy and because their seizures are not under control. Often this anger is directed toward me, their doctor. I can honestly say that I, too, have experienced the emotion of anger at times, and even resentment, especially when patients or their family members, themselves angry and frustrated, demand and expect all my time and insist that I be at their beck and call. It is often difficult for patients and their families to recognize that whereas they are consumed with their own personal situation, their doctor is consumed with the health care of hundreds if not thousands of patients, many of whom are also in desperate trouble.

Still, I have shared in a lot of my patients' joyful occasions—graduations, the purchase of cars, first jobs, marriages, and the births of children. In these instances, it is inevitable that I become sort of an extended family member, because my patients share their successes with me.

Although the emotional reactions that I experience are diverse and sometimes extremely intense, I can't imagine anything else that would give me as much pleasure, as much satisfaction, and as many thrills as when I can favorably improve, by my judgments and decisions, the quality of life for my patients.

26

During my pregraduate studies (before I went into neurology) I had witnessed only one convulsion. I was 14 years old and a boarder in a large institution. At that time we were not given an explanation for what had happened. Instead, for a reason unknown to me, the student who had the seizure was never seen again.

During my neurologic training, I was more impressed by my colleagues than by the patients or their epilepsy. Later on, though, I became fascinated by seizures as the multiple aspects of epilepsy became more evident to me. I was always surprised by seizure descriptions. This aspect of epilepsy still impresses me, even after more than two decades in practice, and more than ever makes me admire how the brain functions.

Another milestone in my growth as a neurologist occurred when a colleague and friend requested that I join the local epilepsy association. It was then that I realized the importance of considering the whole person, not just the seizure description, the diagnostic evaluation, and the treatment plan. Through these experiences, I found that clinicians and patients may have points of view that are as different as the Rocher Percé, the peninsula that Gaspé photographed from two main strategic spots.

Over the years, my expertise in addressing both the clinical and psychosocial aspects of epilepsy has been strengthened by a variety of experiences with many patients. I continue to learn about brain function by analyzing seizure descriptions, and discussing exceptional patients and my personal observations with colleagues always stimulates me.

I believe that these few lines translate the main spikes of my passion for patients and their epilepsy.

27

For about the past year now, my nurse colleagues and I have been working with patients afflicted with intractable seizures. We have been conducting an antiepileptic drug trial on our hospital clinical research unit. This was my first sustained exposure to this patient population in my 6-year career as a nurse. I had witnessed two seizures in the past but I had not been able to identify them as such. Although I feel very comfortable today in caring for my patients with epilepsy, it was a much different story only a year ago.

When we first learned that we were participating in this drug study, I must admit that I was a bit nervous. Nervousness turned into utter panic when it was disclosed that the patients would first be taken off all anticonvulsant medications. I felt that I had to prepare myself to deal with a patient having seizures. The bottom line was that I had to face my fear of not being able to maintain a totally safe environment for a patient in my care, even though I didn't realize this fact for the first few months of the drug trial.

I prepared myself by viewing some training tapes and reading the informational materials provided by our epilepsy nurse specialist. I learned to classify seizures and to understand different aspects of the disorder. I knew that epilepsy wasn't a disease—our nurse specialist had quickly corrected me on this point at our first meeting.

However, all this new knowledge did little to alleviate my fears. I was still shaking in my boots! So I was advised to attend a day-long seminar on epilepsy being presented by our state epilepsy association. Fortunately, I agreed to go, because one of the lectures finally broke the ice. The speaker showed a video of several patients having seizures. Watching the seizure video and listening to the lecturer's description of the stages of the seizures seemed to help my anxiety. I was able to observe the seizures in a nonthreatening way. This teaching tool was truly helpful to me.

As we got ready to receive our first study patient, my colleagues and I were all on edge. Working with the first few patients seemed like baptism by fire, but we all survived. It took me months to be merely uneasy (rather than petrified) when my patient was alone in the bathroom or the shower. I slowly realized that these are everyday normal events for patients, even if they do have a seizure disorder and are surrounded by porcelain.

I found that my initial fears of being unable to guarantee safety for my patients, even in a protected environment, paled in comparison to the courage these people have. In the end it was the patients themselves who brought me to my current level of comfort with seizures.

28

As a licensed clinical social worker, putting into words my feelings about working with patients with seizure disorders has seemed like an insurmountable task. How do I write about my feelings and experiences, and about the rewards of working so closely with such a unique and special group of people? I suppose by starting at the very beginning.

Several years ago my first patient with intractable seizures was referred to me. The referral was made so that I could provide him support for his nonmedical problems. I had prepared for this moment by reviewing pertinent articles and undergoing specialized formal training. I learned about many of the psychosocial issues related to epilepsy, including the restrictions on driving and the problems with unemployment, societal discrimination, memory and cognitive difficulties, mood swings, and medication side effects. But what I didn't know was what it was really like to live with a seizure disorder. I was about to find out.

When my first patient arrived I could feel my heart racing. I had trouble conducting a comprehensive evaluation because I was too focused on his gestures, movements, and breathing. I feared that at any moment he was going to have a seizure. This threat was almost palpable to me and heightened my anxiety and, I suspect, my patient's anxiety level as well. Getting to know who this person was, what he wanted, and what he needed was masked by this pervasive threat. He then proceeded to tell me the indignity that he felt when in fact this threat became reality.

My patient's openness provided me with my first real insight into living with a seizure disorder. I found myself fascinated by his courage. We all need to learn how to cope with the uncertainties of life, but rarely is this uncertainty with us each and every day from the moment we awake. It is for people with epilepsy.

With the support of many wonderful colleagues and special patients, I have gained confidence and knowledge of the medical and personal implications of living with a seizure disorder. More important, I have developed tremendous respect for my patients' abilities to persevere and to cope with and conquer many obstacles.

My initial goal in working with patients is to help them become more comfortable with the daily threat of having a seizure. Only then can they begin to move toward self-awareness and self-identity. Inherent in this goal is the establishment of trust. Meaningful relationships are based on trust. This is often a difficult task in a society that still clings to the mystique of epilepsy. Education has helped to destroy some of the antiquated myths and beliefs, but we have a long way to go. Therefore, perseverance holds a special meaning for these patients because they must still contend with societal myths and prejudices.

Patients need to learn when it feels right for them to disclose their epilepsy to others in a social or employment setting; to take advantage of, rather than to resent the need for, accommodations at work;

to use memory aids; and to be mindful of possible harmful situations. They also need to believe that a suitable workplace is one that provides satisfaction not just for the employer but also for the employee. They need to allow themselves to explore their own strengths, talents, hopes, and dreams in a comfortable, safe, and productive environment.

What began as a difficult task for me has actually proved to be a therapeutic experience. Many years and hundreds of patients later, I continue to be rewarded. My early fascination with the courage of patients with epilepsy has grown into deep admiration, which has stimulated me to extend my work into the community and to help develop community programs and support groups.

I continue to work with individuals and families, and I have seen the achievements and contributions of many wonderful human beings—mothers, fathers, brothers, sisters, professionals, students, workers, and employers.

And oh, yes, most of these people have epilepsy, to.

29

Seizures may take only a few minutes each month, but they can have major consequences.

When I was a neurology resident, epilepsy clinic was held on Fridays. This clinic was not popular with most of my fellow residents because the hours were long, it was extremely busy, the patients had a reputation for being needier than other clinic patients, and most of all it occurred on Friday afternoons! As I look back on how I interacted with the patients in that clinic, I'm struck with how uniform my approach was, regardless of each patient's special situation or the circumstances that may have brought him or her to the clinic. My questions were predictable and always the same: How old are you? When did your seizures begin? How many seizures have you had in the past day, week, month, year? How long do they last? When was the last time you had a seizure? Do your seizures occur in the morning, afternoon, or night? When? How long? How many? Day? Night?

It seemed as though I was keeping some type of seizure scorecard. Time was the central theme in my approach, and decisions about treatment were based on the statistics. Epilepsy, I recall thinking at the time, was a singular condition much like asthma or diabetes, and only a limited number of medications were available to try. All patients were to be put through the same paces. All patients with seizures were the same, and epilepsy was the same for all.

A few years went by, both good and bad clinical experiences accumulated, the angst of being a resident diminished, and I had a little more time to listen to my patients' responses to the questions that I posed. My approach changed and became more individualized.

These days, as I muse over the answers that patients give now to the same inquiries I've always asked, it's interesting to note that the concept of time is still a core issue. Those who experience seizures perceive their events as quite brief. "My seizures last about 1 minute, 2 minutes tops. They're not a big deal." Then, head shaking, the patient's wife, husband, or significant other will quietly interject, "They last 15 to 20 minutes, maybe an hour." The disparity in their answers has always fascinated me. Why is it that the same event experienced by one person but witnessed by many is interpreted differently by all? Investigators have shown that a typical seizure lasts about 1 minute, yet few people ever seem to give that answer; it's always much longer (particularly for observers) or much shorter (especially for the patient).

But there's more to epilepsy than just the duration of seizures. If a reductionist were to define epilepsy as a disease only in terms of the time involved with seizures, he would not consider epilepsy debilitating. Take, for example, the argument presented separately to me by a junior resident and by an insurance reviewer. Each said, "If a patient has four seizures a month and each seizure lasts 1 minute with 5 minutes of postictal confusion, then the total time the patient is affected by epilepsy adds up to only 24 minutes a month. Moreover, only 4 of those 24 minutes are actually spent having seizures. How bad can 24 minutes a month be? That's equivalent to a half-hour comedy show on TV, not counting commercials." When viewed in this manner, epilepsy becomes a mere nuisance, drudgery, or something to get through, like a dental appointment or tax time. There must be a missing element in this contention.

The missing point, of course, is the devastating consequence of those 4 minutes a month of seizures. For a good analogy, look no further than the title of this book, *Brainstorms*. In many ways, people with epilepsy are victims of natural events, just like people who survive tornadoes or earthquakes. In each of those natural events, an unpredictable energy forces the affected person to take cover and to deal later with the aftermath. Earthquakes and tornadoes last only minutes, yet people that live in areas prone to these events spend most of their lives preparing for those fleeting moments.

Four minutes a month shakes the world around people with epilepsy. Society looks at them differently, their friends are more cautious, and activities that had been taken for granted, such as driving, working, and leaving home, all take on a very different perspective and often become impossible.

It's curious how a 1-minute seizure can have such major consequences in a person's life. Consider a taxi driver, cook, or machinist who seeks evaluation for epilepsy. Even if the person has one or two seizures per month, they are the main focus of the person's concern. These patients may take one or more medications, and some may even contemplate brain surgery to prevent further occurrence of these seizures. For these patients, life is radically altered by these relatively rare events.

However, two seizures a month for other patients is nothing short of a blessing. Consider, for example, the person living in a protected, structured environment who in addition to seizures has several other maladies from either a previous head trauma, a difficult birth, or a chronic neurologic condition. These patients are typically accompanied by a case worker at their medical visits and commonly have daily seizures. For them, having two seizures a month is almost always perceived as a positive development and as an indication that their epilepsy is under good control.

How can this be? One person is devastated and the other is seemingly content. Obviously, epilepsy is not the singular condition with features common to all patients that I cavalierly used to think it was as a resident. Like other natural events, such as earthquakes or tornadoes, there is a capriciousness in a seizure's ability to wreak havoc or not, all depending on the situation.

Many years have elapsed since my days as a resident in Friday afternoon epilepsy clinic. Now I supervise neurology residents in a similar setting. The day of the week has changed (it's now Thursday afternoon) but the hours are still long, the patients are just as needy, and the medical questions remain the same.

The difference is that I've come to realize that epilepsy is a unique disorder because of its personalized, individual nature. Whereas other medical problems can be very similar in their presentation and consequences no matter who has these conditions, epilepsy is as distinctive as the person who has it. Unlike other disabilities, it is a condition that is not readily apparent to the outside world. One cannot quickly identify persons who have epilepsy simply by observing them out in the world, but their identity is unmistakable should a seizure occur. Some persons with epilepsy embrace their seizures, some allow their fear of seizures to dictate their lives, and others fight their condition valiantly; each person with epilepsy defines the disorder in his or her own terms.

So now when a neurology resident presents an epilepsy clinic patient with a seizure scorecard, I stop and encourage the resident to consider the major consequences of those few minutes each month.

30

During their training, physicians tend to form stereotypical notions about the typical presentation of particular illnesses and the characteristics of patients with those illnesses. These stereotypes are colored by those who initially teach us and are further biased by our initial personal exposure to an illness, whether it affects a patient in the hospital or a family member or friend.

After I went into practice, it wasn't long before I realized that seizures came in all shapes and sizes. They were far more diverse than the stereotype I had formed in medical school. Many patients with epilepsy present a straightforward picture, whereas others exhibit surprisingly unexpected manifestations of the condition. Although patients with epilepsy comprise an extremely diverse group, many professionals, even those at academic centers, still tend to generalize and to associate all patients with specific dysfunctional characteristics.

A valuable lesson that I have learned is "never say never." Always remember how variable seizures can be. I witnessed the tremendous emotional upheaval of a young woman with chronic, intractable frontal lobe epilepsy who, for many years previously, had been mistakenly labeled with a psychiatric diagnosis and the diagnosis of pseudoseizure. If her doctors had been asked whether she had epilepsy, they would have replied "Never." This experience has helped me to maintain an open mind when the diagnosis of pseudoseizure is considered.

I have also come to realize the tremendous challenges that a patient with epilepsy faces. Few other disorders can attack an otherwise healthy person so often and so unexpectedly, leaving him or her with a life of multiple restrictions and constant threats. Moreover, few of us truly realize the magnitude of the daily issues faced by someone with seizures who tries to maintain a functional lifestyle despite experiencing physical limitations and misguided psychological labels.

Working in the field of epilepsy has been a rewarding and frustrating experience for me. My daily interactions with patients with epilepsy have provided me with many insights into my own life. The most rewarding insight I have gained is a different perspective on the daily activities and responsibilities of life that we usually take for granted. Autonomy, independence, good health, and the realization of our own potential are integral components of our lives that we should all cherish.

31

Mr. Y was admitted to the Epilepsy Clinic when he was 15 years old. He had frequent tonic–clonic seizures and myoclonic jerks. A diffuse tremor affected his arms and disturbed his voice. He walked with difficulty because of impaired balance. The diagnosis of myoclonic epilepsy was made, and he received trials of several different drugs.

Mr. Y continued to be seen as an outpatient at the epilepsy center at least once a year. He lived with his mother a thousand kilometers from our clinic. Since they were poor, they took the train. Each trip to and from the center took at least 2 days and caused considerable expense for the family. All this effort for a 20-minute examination and one routine EEG tracing!

Fortunately, Mr. Y's seizure frequency progressively decreased and, recently, his seizures finally stopped. However, he continued to have trouble walking and had almost continuous tremors. We began to explain the severity of his illness to him and the likelihood that he would never recover enough to lead a normal life. He understood that prospect very well.

Overall, though, Mr. Y did much better over the years. When he was 30 years old I tried to increase the time between his clinic visits and proposed that he return for a checkup every 2 years. We could intermingle the visits with telephone contact and even possibly refer him to a medical center closer to his home. He became upset about this proposal and refused to discuss the matter further. He got up and left the room, sobbing.

We were amazed because we believed that, if anything, our suggestion would have been reassuring to him. His mother tried to explain her son's behavior: "He is fully aware of his condition, and he is not afraid of it. He knows he must take medication for the rest of his life, that he cannot get a job, and that it will be hard for him to have friends. He knows that for him to dream of having a family with a wife and kids is forbidden. He is strong, and in fact he sometimes tries to solve *my* troubles. But sorry, Doctor, you said something that he cannot accept, something that sounds as if you are abandoning him to his fate. I know that you did this for us, but our problems don't matter. He *wants* and *needs* to come here and talk to you for a while. This is important to him. Please, give us an appointment for next year."

We doctors have to keep in mind that 5 minutes more of our precious time may immensely help our patients, even if there are no decisions to be made. I told Mr. Y nothing he did not already know. It was up to him, that time, to teach me something of invaluable importance that *I* didn't know.

32

I had been in private practice only a few months when I met a gentle, unassuming man named Bob. He had a powerful sense of confidence in me. Although he was 3 years younger than I, we had many things in common. Like my wife and me, Bob and his wife were expecting a second child soon. As in my case, he had graduated from a university with a bright future before him. Unlike me, however, Bob began to have complex partial seizures (CPS) and to suffer cognitive impairment caused by the seizures and by the medications required to minimize them.

Bob worked as a school custodian and a newspaper delivery man. His wife, a former teacher, was a devoted homemaker and sold household supplies part time. They eventually bought a house and had two lovely children. Although Bob was happy with his life, he wanted me to help him become seizure-free.

At the age of 15 months, Bob had had a prolonged febrile convulsion. Later, his seizures failed to come under control despite trials of a number of different seizure medications used in various combinations. After my initial visit with him he underwent a sleep EEG which, for the first time, revealed left temporal lobe epileptiform discharges. I added a new seizure medication to the three drugs he was already taking. I was pleased because he subsequently had no CPS for over 6 months and resumed driving for the first time in years.

Unfortunately, the medications made Bob tired and irritable. I began to taper off some of his original medications. When his regimen had been reduced to only two drugs, he felt better but his CPS returned. Eventually his seizure control improved and Bob again resumed driving. One day, after missing a morning dose of medication, he had a CPS but nevertheless got in his car. While he was driving on an interstate highway, he had another CPS, which caused a car accident. After this experience, despite several other very high-dose medication trials, his CPS continued at a rate of seven to eight seizures a month. Bob gave up driving.

I really wanted to help Bob. Deep in my heart I believed that it would probably take surgery to stop his seizures, but of course we first needed to give all the available medications a chance.

Bob was highly motivated to be rid of his seizures and was very compliant with office visits and medication trials. With this in mind, I recommended that he undergo video/EEG monitoring. The results would determine whether he was a candidate for surgery. I had just started a new epilepsy center and surgical program at that time. Bob put his trust in me. The testing indicated that surgery might help him, and he gladly became one of the first patients to be operated on at our new center.

Since then, Bob has been seizure-free and is on a lower dose of just a single seizure medication. He drives, has much more energy at home and at work, is no longer moody, and thinks more clearly. Neuropsychologic testing confirmed that his IQ improved after the surgery.

Of all my patients, Bob remains most vivid in my memory. Why? In part because he was one of the first patients at our center whose epilepsy was treated successfully with surgery. However, it was also because of his confidence that I could help him become seizure-free. His confidence in me motivated me to keep working until we achieved his goal. It took 3 years and the use of four drugs to obtain reasonably good seizure control, but that control came at the price of sedation and moodiness. I believed that Bob was a great candidate for surgery, and it turned out I was right. Brain surgery intimidates most patients, and Bob was no exception. Good rapport had been established between us from his frequent visits over 3 years, and I was able to reassure him and allay his concerns. He sailed through surgery, and I felt enormous satisfaction from having helped this confident young man take his first steps toward achieving his dreams, free from the seizure disorder that had held him back for over 30 years.

Bob's confidence and the outcome of his surgery continue to motivate me, years later, to search out and help similar patients. My wife and I still get Christmas cards from his family.

33

What are some of the many emotions I have felt while working with people with epilepsy? Helplessness, sadness, inadequacy, frustration, empathy, compassion, anger, joy, connectedness, responsibility, thankfulness, gratefulness, fear, and hope. Although my experiences are not always pleasant, I cherish them all and am grateful for what patients have taught me. Let me share a few stories with you.

David came for a follow-up visit last week. He said that things were as usual. He was having seizures that made him fall and injure himself about every other day, in spite of all the treatments we had recommended. He mentioned, with little emotion, some of the accidents he had recently had. And then he spoke about his daughter's graduation. He had experienced a seizure during the ceremony, despite doing everything he knew to try to prevent it from happening. He was asked to leave. After he recovered from the seizure, he was almost barred from returning because people thought he was drunk. He expressed how awful he felt because his daughter had a dad like him. I felt so helpless, so inadequate, and so sad for both of them.

Another of my patients, Cheryl, coached me in really slow speech before I went to give a talk in Texas. "You know, when you go down South, you better get used to people speaking very slowly." Cheryl died a year ago. I can still feel her smile and the place she had in my heart. And it still hurts. I miss her a lot.

At a recent meeting about epilepsy, I ran into 50-year-old Joe and his parents, who still care for him and his epilepsy. We had lunch together during the meeting break. A few days later, I received a wonderful note from Joe's mother, thanking me for joining them at lunch. I am grateful to her for reminding me that little things, things that I take for granted, do matter to others. And I thank them for raising my awareness about the importance of communication and interaction.

Janice had experienced seizures since childhood. In addition to seizures, she had several other problems. We felt quite successful because we were able to control her seizures and migraines with delicate management of several medications. Then Janice called to tell me that "things weren't all right." She was frustrated more than ever because she didn't have a job that she liked.

My initial reaction was disappointment and anger. Somehow I thought that she should at least be a bit satisfied with the improvement in her symptoms. I guess I expected her to be grateful. But then I realized, yet again, that we had not been able to achieve what mattered most to *her*, which was to be gainfully employed in a meaningful job and to live an independent life. How much of this was my responsibility? And what could *I* do?

Sometimes, when my own fear of developing a chronic condition gets to me, I run the danger of dealing with it the way I deal with war—I tend to protect myself by thinking that it happens far away, to other faceless strangers.

Susan took me right out of that illusion. She bluntly asked, "What would you do if you couldn't drive? How would you get to work? How would you live on $70 a week?" I didn't have answers to her questions. And I realized that I had never considered the possibilities, either. I felt arrogant for assuming that I would never have to face those problems.

Yesterday, a friend mentioned that she thought I was courageous because I was determined to do things that scared me. I thought of Susan and how much courage she mounted every day in her uphill battle to work and live independently. I feel guilty for having so many options and frustrated about the inequalities in our society that reward my enterprises in overcoming fear but that don't reward hers as easily. Thanks to Susan, I was humbled. I respect her very much for her boldness.

Because a new combination of medicines was tried, Michael's seizures during the past year were under much better control. However, both he and his fiancée had been nervous about the possibility that Michael would have a seizure during their upcoming wedding ceremony. So we decided that he should take an extra pill to relax him on the day of the wedding if he felt that he needed it.

We talked about Michael's medications during his visit after the wedding. He had a big smirk on his face. It turned out that he had felt confident enough in himself and in the control of his seizures that he did not think he needed the extra medicine and did not take it. He was very proud of his success. As I sit here writing about our last encounter, I smile at his confidence and can still feel his joy.

People with epilepsy have taught me many lessons, personally and professionally. First, medical care is only one part of their lives. Second, many things that I take for granted and at times forget about really do matter. Third, I may not be able to change society, but I can at least be a piece in the mosaic of my patients' lives, if sometimes only by listening actively.

I am extremely grateful to my patients with epilepsy for helping me grow, with compassion, every day.

34

Last Christmas, one of my patients gave me a gift that she had made herself. It was a needlepoint design of a small lighthouse on a deserted beach. The present took me by surprise. Over the previous 2 years we had tried everything to control her seizures, but nothing had helped her very much. If anything, her seizures were worse. She told me she wanted me to know that she appreciated what I was doing for her, because I wouldn't give up on her.

In my neurology practice I see only patients with epilepsy. I have been doing this for a number of years and have treated over one thousand patients. I chose epilepsy as my specialty for two reasons, one academic, the other practical. First, the functional anatomy of the brain has fascinated me since I was a student. I knew that trying to understand how the brain works could challenge me enough for an entire career. Second, as a practicing physician I wanted to take care of people I could really help. During my neurology residency, it appeared as though we couldn't do much for patients with most neurologic diseases, such as muscular dystrophy, stroke, or dementia. But epilepsy patients were dramatically different. Once a correct diagnosis was made and the proper medication was prescribed, seizures could be stopped. I was lucky to learn from teachers who were experts in treating epilepsy. Patients came from all over the world to see them. I saw that many people with epilepsy had their seizures completely controlled, and almost all of them experienced significant improvement. Sometimes epilepsy surgery actually cured someone.

I did a fellowship in electroencephalography because I liked the idea of studying brain waves and learning how to identify an epileptic focus. Now I apply my technical expertise to help people with epilepsy control their seizures.

One might think that the patients I remember best are those with the most successful outcomes, the ones whose seizures vanished. But that's not true. The way things work, I rarely have time to think about the patients who do well. I see patients only about once a year after their seizures come under control. When they do come to the office, the visits are pleasant but usually brief. I refill their prescriptions, we smile and shake hands, and they're gone for another year.

It is the patients with recurrent seizures whom I remember best because I see them again and again every few weeks. I find their charts on my desk with notes from the on-call physician describing yet another side effect, an injury from a seizure, or a visit to the emergency room. Their clinic visits are long and arduous. I listen to their tales of frustration about not being able to drive. Their faces are grim, and sometimes I sense anger in their voices when they tell me about another job lost because of a seizure. They list their epilepsy medications and struggle to remember the dosages. Many take an antidepressant, and with good reason. Together we grope for answers. Is there an anticonvulsant we haven't tried? Should we experiment with an investigational drug? Should we consider brain surgery, even if it only stops most but not all of the seizures?

For some patients with difficult-to-control epilepsy, our cooperative struggle against their seizures yields worthwhile results. We reduce medications from three to two and then to one. Seizures decrease from twice a week to twice a month. Side effects diminish. Phone calls taper off. The visits become shorter and less frequent. For other patients, piles of seizure calendars, anticonvulsant drug levels, and dictated notes accumulate. Their charts grow into behemoths and threaten to explode at the seams. Bottle after bottle of expensive drugs with exotic names, telephone calls with complaints of dizziness, hospitalizations for epilepsy monitoring, and innumerable office visits do not seem to get us anywhere. Yet we continue to try. We know that without the medications the seizures would be worse.

Each year I attend the American Epilepsy Society meeting. Investigators from around the world present the results of hundreds of research projects. I reassure my patients that millions of dollars and many of the world's finest scientific minds are devoted to understanding their disorder. There *will* be therapeutic advances. Next year, or the year after, we *will* have something else to try. And this time, it just might work.

What reassures *me* is the picture of the lighthouse on my wall, symbolic of what our patients unselfishly give us and what we can give to them in return.

The beacon is burning. The promise of progress illuminates the night.

35

The director of an epilepsy clinic referred Stuart, an adolescent with Lennox–Gastaut syndrome, to me. The neurologist knew that I, as a child psychiatrist and family therapist, used a family-based approach in working with young people. But I knew that I had little previous experience with epilepsy. In fact, I could barely recall my medical school lectures on epilepsy, so I looked the syndrome up in one of my medical texts. I learned that Lennox–Gastaut syndrome affected cognition and produced a variety of seizures that were almost impossible to treat. We were up against a formidable enemy.

Stuart was referred because a disastrous series of seizures had threatened what remained of his normal life and devastated his coping abilities. He was failing with peers and schoolwork, and he had difficulty living up to his family's expectations. He was slowly spiraling toward depression.

As I started working with Stuart, I discovered that he believed there was a conspiracy against him. I think he adopted this belief to protect himself from a reality that he found very frightening. He believed that he was part of a motorcycle gang that was in the midst of pulling off a major drug deal. In this scenario, all the danger of his life with epilepsy remained but his macho belief in himself was preserved. His fear was focused on something other than his seizures. When asked about his seizures, he simply said, "When the going gets tough, the tough get going."

I also met with Stuart's family—his mother, father, and sisters—and felt their despair, confusion, and anxiety about his medical condition and the strange beliefs he had begun to report to them. I felt as overwhelmed as they did. Stuart, in turn, was worried about his family because he feared that there might be an attack against them. Needless to say, his epilepsy had attacked everyone.

Stuart's delusional beliefs compounded the side effects of medications, the severe and devastating impact of seizures on his body and spirit, the difficulty he had establishing independence and self-esteem, and the fears and sadness of his family. No wonder everyone longed for the answer.

How could I remain centered as Stuart's therapist and still be open to the terrible pain that he and his family were experiencing? How could I help him focus on and manage his medical fears, as well as the imaginary ones he had created, when his mind was swirling in an epileptic storm? His seizures diminished the very resources he needed to rally. He was tired, irritable, and sleep-deprived. He was angry whenever he was hospitalized "for the stupid seizures that the hospital didn't help anyway." I became his designated psychological helper, a role that he perceived as indicating that he had failed. More stigma for him to bear.

Along with Stuart and his family, I was reeling from these complex issues. I could barely catch my breath as they shared their valiant efforts to restore a sense of normalcy to their day-to-day lives. I needed to find a perspective that permitted me to admire their extraordinary efforts and enabled them to discuss their raw emotional pain. I had to help them strengthen their resources and let them share their feelings about their struggle.

My work required me to move within the experiential realm of Stuart and his parents. Before I could help them address their many problems, there were enormous layers of feelings for me to identify and manage. Only then could I recognize the internal barriers that they created to wall off their most intense feelings, intense feelings caused by Stuart's mind-altering and physically intrusive disorder and that had to be aired.

I eventually found a perspective that enabled me to communicate and acknowledge their pain. Even as Stuart's physical well-being was threatened by many devastating drop attacks, his parents remained courageous. I came to accept my own powerlessness over their many emotional traumas. As their struggles and discussions in therapy helped to reestablish a foundation for coping, I felt strengthened by their resolve and knew that progress would be made.

Perhaps because of my experiences with Stuart and his family, I began to work more and more with families assaulted by epilepsy. In the course of this work I often had discussions with family members concerning their reactions to grand mal seizures. Ironically I had never personally witnessed one and could not have predicted how complex and intimate *my* emotional response to this type of seizure would be. Until I saw one.

Benjamin, his parents, and I had returned to their home after an extended meeting at Benjamin's school. Benjamin had also received a diagnosis of Lennox–Gastaut syndrome and had experienced frequent major motor seizures. We were chatting in the living room when Benjamin appeared in the frame of the kitchen doorway. We watched as he approached us and suddenly dropped. As he hit the floor I experienced a variety of feelings: surprise, confusion, fear, feelings of being overwhelmed and of being suspended in time, awe, sadness, and a longing to change what was happening.

Emotions in the room instantly rose to a nearly unbearable level. Benjamin's mother's stifled cry was audible in the sudden silence, and she dropped to the floor next to Benjamin to cradle his head in her lap. His father's face showed anxiety and surprise.

I was left standing, still helpless, confused, surprised, frightened, and saddened. As Benjamin lay there and I began to recover from the emotional shock of watching him seize, I realized that his father was distancing himself from becoming involved. As his facial expression changed to an impassive grimace, he gradually backed out of the room and went upstairs to his private quarters.

Benjamin's mother had long ago mastered the role of preventing her son from becoming injured by a seizure. Her anguish was obvious, yet she was by his side, protecting his thrashing body. Her husband could deal with his feelings in this situation only by isolating himself from his son. Other fathers might have used their power and influence to advocate for their child, but not Benjamin's father. I finally understood how difficult it would be for me to master my feelings under these circumstances. How would I react if my own child had grand mal seizures?

Benjamin's seizure stopped abruptly, but its emotional impact diminished more slowly. As had happened many times before, his family gradually regrouped and reaffirmed their plans, goals, and hopes for Benjamin. They all felt that he could move further toward an independent life. That he *would* do it. I admired them for enduring the epileptic attack and redirecting their energy in a positive direction toward recovery.

I have also been impressed by how that energy can be misdirected at other times. Denise was in therapy with me during her late adolescence and young adulthood. She had poorly controlled partial complex seizures that occasionally became secondarily generalized. Our confrontational meetings about her cocaine abuse, her relationships with risky young men, and how she got her family to cover her tracks when she dropped the ball eventually enabled her to stabilize and become involved in a recovery program.

During one particularly stressful session, Denise focused on the intense loss she felt after ending a relationship with someone who had never respected her. She had always felt inadequate and afraid of managing her own affairs. We agreed that her ex-boyfriend was like a drug with horrible side effects. Denise admitted that in his presence she forgot her own fears and concerns. As she recalled this loss and the moments of intense conflict that preceded their breakup, her emotions intensified and she suddenly had a strange look in her eyes. She said that she was beginning to have a seizure. I knew that her seizures were occasionally triggered by intense emotion.

As the seizure intensified, her consciousness became clouded and we lost contact. Then, rhythmic jerking started in her right arm and began to spread. I found myself thinking, "Oh, my God, I need to get a doctor!" This experience reminded me how overpowering a seizure can be to an observer. That thought was followed by the flash realization that *I* was the doctor. I knew as well as Benjamin's mother what to do in this situation and rapidly took action. I helped her move from the chair to the floor, but her head fell back and began to knock against the wall. I moved her and kept her on her side to protect her from hitting the furniture. Confusion, fear, surprise, helplessness, loss: it all came back to me yet again.

I knew that all the feelings welling up in me would need to be addressed and managed by Denise so that she could to live among other people who might witness her seizures. Managing other people's feelings about epilepsy often proves to be as challenging to the person with seizures as managing the illness!

The ways in which children with epilepsy struggle to understand their world is captivating. The personal encouragement I feel as they master the dilemmas presented to them by their seizures is very rewarding. One memorable example was my work with Teddy. He was 4 years old when we met and had already had recurrent, brief visual seizures for over a year.

Teddy's astute parents had called these episodes "flashes" to help their son label what was happening within him. However, Teddy's delayed language development prevented him from grasping this idea with words. As a result, much of our communication during therapy sessions occurred through play. Teddy used light switches to bring his world of flashing lights into the playroom. When he improvised uncontrollable and terrifying storms, we huddled together under an umbrella. As his seizures progressed, elements of fear and more complex, mysterious visual impressions entered his play. Gradually, he became preoccupied with the beginning of this new seizure: a dark figure in his visual flash.

Vampires, Darth Vader, black capes, and masks became part of Teddy's world and, in turn, the playroom. He tried to become what he feared so that he would fear it less. Better to try to be a monster than to feel vulnerable to being attacked by one. The degree of fear he associated with these episodes was profound. He began to ask questions about what was real and what was unreal. Struggling to sort out what had affected his life, he would ask repeatedly what around him was dead. Was he dead? Was I dead? How did things get to be dead or undead?

What could or would stop these episodes? Teddy's play included scenarios in which nothing could stop Darth Vader or the Vampires. No super-hero, no Mom or Dad, no valiant fellow could stop that dark shadow. He was right—there was no rescue from those moments. Medicine had helped, but the flashes and longer seizures were still there. As his therapist, I had to tolerate those basic questions for which there were few answers.

Teddy had to learn that he could endure these terrible episodes without dying. Even if Mom or Dad, the doctors, or I could not make these episodes go away, we could still help him. Once again I faced my own limitations but dug deep into my understanding, knowledge, and belief in what a therapist can offer those who struggle against pain and failure. Together with his parents, I tried to work out a way to help him understand his seizures and a way to support and reassure him.

Little by little, Teddy established a real sense of control and learned how to define his competence. It didn't mean that everything was better or that significant handicaps were no longer present, but rather that his tools to manage the difficulties were in the best shape possible.

My experiences with Stuart, Benjamin, Denise, and Teddy underscore the reasons why I have valued working with people facing the enormous challenges of epilepsy. My faith and optimism have been constantly validated by my work, even in the midst of bleak times. Although I have now witnessed many different types of seizures, I must confess that I still feel the same range of emotions every time. All aspects of a person's being—personal vitality, presence, and physical well-being—are taken over by the seizure. I feel that the connection to the person is lost at that moment. This sense of loss reminds me of the loss and sadness associated with life itself.

Seeing the inner strengths that persons with epilepsy discover as they successfully face their challenges has encouraged me. As someone said at a recent conference, the path for someone with epilepsy may be a long and hard one but it should lead to constructive denial, not debilitating acceptance. Finding the right balance between acceptance and detachment is like a walking a tightrope. Complex feelings accompany seizures, even when the seizure symptoms occur only in the mind of the patient. To emotionally support a patient and his or her family, I must see how these tremendously intense and internal feelings reverberate in everyone.

The courage and adaptiveness of the human spirit displayed by people with epilepsy have sustained my own spirit and energy. Sharing the dilemmas of the emotional roller coaster that is epilepsy has reaffirmed my commitment to therapeutic work. I will continue to help people gain the confidence they need to develop honest and supportive relationships with family members, members of their communities, and their circle of friends.

In my own life, the importance of sharing has become a touchstone. And now, when someone with epilepsy gives me that look that says, "Did you know that I just had a seizure?" I know the issue is that we *both* know, and we have to get back to work!

36

I have worked exclusively with patients with epilepsy for almost 22 years. Now, when I look back at my early experiences, I realize how very little I knew then about this very complex disorder.

At the beginning of my career, the extensive training and education that I received about the medical aspects of epilepsy prepared me to understand the disorder from the academic perspective. However, the knowledge I have acquired over the years about the challenges and consequences of epilepsy has come from patients, their families, their friends and, sometimes, from their teachers and employers.

I am struck by the diverse nature of this disorder. I have learned that seizure freedom alone does not guarantee a normal, productive life. I have seen, for example, physically impaired persons with uncontrolled seizures who manage to complete their education, function well in jobs, get married, and raise families. I have also seen physically healthy people with well-controlled seizures who are overwhelmingly handicapped by the diagnosis of epilepsy and who have inadequate, poorly learned coping skills.

Our patients and their families need to realize that the key to a healthy, productive life is rather complex and that it depends on many other factors in addition to becoming seizure-free.

37

Several years ago, some time before I began working as a secretary in an epilepsy clinic, I met one of our patients in a coffee bar. I was sitting at a small table alone reading a literary magazine and drinking an extra large cup of java and feeling as if I did not have a care in the world. This particular table had a bad habit of tipping on its pedestal and, consequently, I splashed some coffee onto the table. When I got up for a napkin, the young man sitting at the table across from me started speaking to me from across the room.

He told me how lonely life was for "someone like him" and wondered why he did not have a girlfriend like everyone else his age. Although I did not know what he meant by his self-description of "someone like me," I knew that he was speaking from the bottom of his heart. I concurred that life was indeed very lonely at times. "What should I do?" he asked. I said, "I don't know" and asked him if he ever went to church. "No," he said. He was raised a Catholic but no longer attended Mass. I mentioned that the church I attended had a young people's group for people in their twenties and that he would be welcome to join in their activities whether he was interested in attending church or not. In fact, some people from the group would be going on an overnight trip in a few weeks.

The young man appeared very discouraged at the thought of any social interaction at all, and he seemed unwilling to reveal anything more about himself. We said our good-byes, and I did not see him again until I began working in the epilepsy clinic. Neither of us has ever acknowledged that we met previously.

Now, when I call to remind the same young man of an upcoming appointment, his new girlfriend often answers the phone. Perhaps that is why, when I see him in the clinic, he seems a bit more hopeful, occasionally even cheerful.

38

I had departed for San Francisco for 5 days of vacation. Leaving one little girl behind in the hospital had made my departure much more difficult. That little girl was my patient Angela, a lovely 6-year-old in whom epilepsy had been diagnosed a year and a half ago. Because all the medication options had been exhausted and her seizures were becoming more frequent and severe, Angela had undergone epilepsy surgery at our center. The neurosurgeon had performed a new procedure: transections of areas that could not be removed safely (because it would have caused permanent weakness).

Most of her abnormal brain tissue had been successfully removed-but the surgery had failed. It was like removing one volcano and trying to plug up another one, only to cause new and more powerful volcanoes to erupt. In more than 200 epilepsy surgery cases performed at our center, this one had been followed by the most unexpected and disappointing result that we had experienced. Some failures are cruel. I had seen fear and pain in Angela's eyes and in her parents' eyes. They didn't understand the medical details but they knew that things were going from bad to worse. As I left for vacation, Angela lay in the intensive care unit, having brief but very distressing seizures every few minutes. She cried and called for her mommy when she wasn't seizing. When she seized, her eyes darted out of control and her left side jerked. A few minutes' rest and then the horrible tape was replayed over and over.

We had tried massive doses of medications in a dizzying array of combinations, but we barely made a dent against the frequency or severity of the attacks for more than several hours at a time. There were no more options for Angela. One more try at surgery was all that was left. The problem was that not only had surgery failed the first time but that it appeared to have made things worse.

Five days of vacation passed in a moment. When I returned to my office on Monday morning I faced the usual avalanche of phone calls, messages from colleagues, and issues concerning the dozen or so inpatients under my care, including several new epilepsy surgery cases. Angela was still in the intensive care unit and was never far from my thoughts. Shackled by the flood of patients, I was unable to spend much time with her and her parents, but I did manage to find time to study her seizures carefully. I kept thinking that this was her last chance.

Two days later Angela returned to surgery. A series of metal electrodes embedded in plastic were placed over her brain to record her seizures and to identify, if possible, where the seizures were coming from. The electrodes could also be used to stimulate her brain with weak electrical currents, to locate motor and sensory areas that could not be safely removed surgically.

Because Angela had seizures every few minutes, the answers came quickly. There was one main seizure focus in an area that could be safely removed, but there was another seizure focus that couldn't be removed without causing leg weakness. To make things worse, several other brain areas showed worrisome activity. My initial fear—that we wouldn't find a focus—had been allayed, but my greater fear persisted, that if we removed one hot spot another one would emerge, as it had the last time she had surgery. What should we do? This young girl's suffering was intense. She had been living in the hospital for 6 weeks with almost continuous seizures.

We held a conference to discuss Angela's case. Because we were so worried about another surgical failure, we changed our approach and converted two-stage surgery into three stages. We removed and transected (the new procedure to limit seizure spread and preserve functional areas) what we could. However, the abnormal activity persisted and it looked nasty. The electrodes were repositioned, and we planned to record her seizures over the weekend. If there were no more seizures over the next couple of days, we would remove the electrodes; otherwise, we would try one last surgical procedure. This additional monitoring would give us one more shot if more volcanoes erupted.

By Sunday we are back where we started. High doses of medications were knocking her out, but every few minutes Angela continued to have seizures coming from the area we couldn't transect. We discussed the possibility of removing the additional area, which would cause lifelong left leg weakness. But the real possibility that inflicting permanent injury would still leave Angela with seizures (from a new hot spot) made this a very difficult choice. By nature I am an optimist, but my optimism was quickly fading.

We decided to recommend additional transections. Angela returned to surgery, and with repositioning there was better access to the area deep in her brain that controlled her left leg muscles. The transections were made in the hot areas and in some other areas that still showed epileptic activity.

It was 6:15 am. Just as Angela was recovering from her third surgery, my associate called. Steve, 19-year-old man with refractory seizures, had recently been started on a new drug. Although his seizures were better controlled on this new drug, high blood pressure developed (possibly from the medication, although his would be the first known case) and antihypertensive treatment was begun. My colleague informed me: "Steve woke in the middle of the night with a headache and then became paralyzed on the left side of his body, unable to speak. He was rushed to a community hospital. His father was screaming over and over that he was going to sue." My heart sank, not because of the threat of a suit (which certainly didn't lift my spirits) but because of what might be happening to Steve, a young man with his entire life in front of him. I had a gut feeling—call it necrologic common sense—that he had bled into his brain.

I was weary. It just didn't seem worth it anymore. "Do no harm" kept echoing in my head. First Angela, now Steve.

Steve was transferred to our hospital. A computed tomography scan showed no blood in his brain, which meant that a stroke was the most likely explanation for his acute illness. However the MRI was perfectly normal, making a stroke unlikely. His speech returned, and his left arm strength improved. His left leg remained weak for several days and he was unable to walk.

The pieces of Steve's picture weren't fitting together. The findings on his examination were inconsistent. Curiously, he did not appear worried or depressed about his weakness. Could he be subconsciously producing this weakness? To answer this question, we injected him with sodium amytal ("truth serum"). His strength returned and he walked. While Steve was under the influence of the amytal, we learned that he was very stressed at work. Conversion disorder, the modern term for hysteria, was the diagnosis. How did stress bring this vigorous young man to unconsciously fake a stroke? Exactly where is that line between consciousness and unconsciousness? Exactly how much do patients with conversion disorder know? What parts of the brain are involved with this disorder? What is the anatomy of the unconscious? These are questions that I often wonder about.

Two weeks later, Angela became seizure-free and was taking less medication. Steve was walking. Appearances are deceiving, frames of reference are traps, common sense is sometimes nonsense, but sleep is great.

Three years later, Steve is fine, but Angela still has intermittent focal motor seizures as we desperately try to reduce her polytherapy.

39

Caring for people with seizures as their nurse has enabled me to share experiences that very few others have been privileged to have. I pride myself in attempting to empower my patients with knowledge that may improve their quality of life. Working through the stigma of having a seizure disorder by discussing the subject often diminishes the patient's anxiety and emotional pain. I am particularly reminded of the wonderful experience I had while caring for a challenging young man, Tom, who was enrolled in an investigational drug study. He was receiving four anticonvulsant drugs when he started the study. He had a number of partial seizures every day and was suffering profound adverse effects.

By the time of Tom's second visit I had serious doubts that we could improve his seizure control. However, as we explored his lifestyle, we found certain habits that were triggering his seizures. His daily intake of caffeine and nicotine was copious, he had irregular sleep habits, and he consumed an unbalanced diet. He had only a few friends at work and otherwise kept himself socially isolated, adding to his level of stress. Near the end of that visit he had a secondarily generalized seizure.

Tom's physician and I decided on a plan to increase his study medication while I began the task of modifying his lifestyle. I started by teaching him what seizure triggers were and how they can influence seizures. Tom was markedly dependent on caffeine and nicotine, using coffee and cigarettes to combat the sedative effects of his anticonvulsants. It was a struggle just to convince him to convert to decaffeinated coffee. We accomplished this goal gradually. After a few additional visits, Tom started using a nicotine patch.

Tom's status had improved so much in a relatively short time that he grew keenly interested in improving the other problem areas of his life. We agreed not to take on too many problems at once so that he would not be overwhelmed by challenges. By the time of his annual visit for the investigational study, Tom was experiencing substantially fewer seizures and was taking better care of himself and feeling more confident. He confided to me that he had even started to date. In light of these encouraging developments, the medical team decided to continue simplifying his anticonvulsant therapy, and I continued to recommend modifications in his lifestyle.

Eventually, Tom became seizure-free on only two anticonvulsants, ceased smoking, was being considered for a promotion at work, and asked a young woman to marry him! I met his fiancée, who expressed her gratitude to me for turning his life around. I felt that I had achieved a wonderful thing by consistently showing him that I cared about him. He was a shining example of what we can do for our patients.

Tom went on to marry his fiancée and they purchased a condo. I believe he is doing well to this day.

40

Karen was 17 when she first came to the clinic. Because of a prolonged febrile seizure she had experienced in childhood, complex partial seizures developed that began with an epigastric sensation and then progressed to oral automatisms and a prolonged postictal state. Her seizures went back as far as she could remember. She had never gone a significant length of time without them, and they had interrupted her schooling and had been an enormous frustration to her. Although Karen looked some years younger than her age, she was nevertheless determined to become more independent, to move away from home, and to be like other young people. Over the next 3 or 4 years we struggled together to find a combination of drugs that might enable her to fulfill her aspirations. She took part in an early clinical trial with one of the new generation of antiepileptic drugs. Her seizures continued to be frequent, and it was unusual for more than a day or two in a row to elapse without her experiencing seizures.

In the mid 1980s our center began to develop a program of surgical treatment for epilepsy. Previously, surgery for epilepsy had been restricted to only two or three centers in the United Kingdom and patients were subjected to extremely long waiting times. When we began our surgical program, Karen expressed an immediate interest despite the concerns and worries of her protective parents.

After the usual presurgical evaluation, Karen was offered and subsequently underwent a right temporal lobectomy. She awoke from her anesthesia with a dense left hemiplegia. She was the sixth patient to undergo temporal lobectomy and the first to experience a serious complication.

The day that Karen returned to the outpatient clinic for the first time after a period of rehabilitation is engraved on my memory. This meeting has probably influenced my approach to people with epilepsy and their management more than any other. Karen walked into the clinic still showing evidence of a moderately severe hemiplegic gait and with a functionally useless left hand. I was a little surprised that she had come to the clinic by herself, as previously she had always attended with her parents.

I began to tell her how sorry I was about the complications of her operation and mumbled some apologies for suggesting it. This was as far as I got. Karen stopped me in the kindest way and pointed out to her uncomprehending doctor that she had been entirely seizure-free since her operation. For the first time she was now able to get on buses by herself and to go out by herself. In effect, she had attained much of the independence to which she had aspired. She expressed the view that moderately severe hemiparesis was much less disabling than frequent complex partial seizures. She explained this in sympathetic terms, as if instructing a small and somewhat naive child.

The realization dawned on me that although I had been treating epilepsy and advising people with the disorder for 10 to 15 years, I had failed to truly understand the nature of the problems facing them in their everyday lives. In Karen's case I had been too quick to impose my own judgments about disability on the results of her surgery. I had spent my clinical life trying to avoid the paternalism that I felt doctors sometimes showed toward many of their patients, only to be as guilty of it as any of my colleagues.

I hope that Karen has taught me to listen more carefully to people with epilepsy and to understand their disability a little better. I certainly feel considerably less qualified to make management decisions on behalf of people with epilepsy, and I endeavor to spend more time presenting information so that they can make their own decisions. I have never had seizures or epilepsy, and I hope I never will. I realize that I will never have a full understanding of its impact.

Karen is now in her early thirties and her doctor is in his early fifties. Unfortunately, after being seizure-free for 3 years, Karen has experienced a return of her seizures, but they are less severe and much less frequent. She remains hemiparetic but enjoys life and has a stable relationship with someone who also has epilepsy.

Strangely, we both benefitted in different ways, in spite of, in Karen's case, and because of, in my case, a medical accident.

41

Each day as I enter our epilepsy unit, I reflect upon one of the darkest times in my life, one that created a special bond between my patients and me.

Two years ago I found myself in the waiting room of the intensive care unit, not in my role as a physician but instead as a husband. The same respirator that had been used before to support the breathing of my patients with uncontrolled seizures was now sustaining the life of my comatose and paralyzed wife, herself a physician, in whom a devastating pulmonary illness had developed.

Suddenly, as my role changed from that of a health-care provider to family member, I was ordered to leave my wife's room. I was accustomed to providing answers to my patients, but now I found myself worried that I would bother my wife's doctor by asking too many questions. In what was a previously unimaginable switch, it was now I, the physician, who was anxious, tearful, and receiving cards and words of support from patients.

Perhaps it is impossible to truly understand the overwhelming feelings that serious illness engenders until one has been personally touched by it. Words used by my patients with epilepsy such as *fear*, *depression*, and *anxiety* began to have new meaning for me in light of my wife's illness. Even the anger that well-intentioned physicians occasionally encounter in their patients became more understandable to me. Although my wife was awake, she was unable to move or speak, but only rarely did anyone ever try to communicate with her, to understand her needs, or to explain to her what was happening. Although I was extremely grateful for the superb medical care she received, I felt helpless and exasperated when the staff did not immediately respond to problems, and I worried about what was happening when I couldn't be there. When I had to leave her to attend to the neglected aspects of my life, such as our two young children at home, it made me feel guilty and as though I were abandoning her.

With a few rare exceptions, I was also deeply disturbed to find that most of the compassion expressed directly to my wife came not from doctors but rather from nurses, clergy, technicians, and housekeeping staff. It occurred to me that there must be something terribly wrong with a medical education system that fails to nurture the capacity of physicians to relate emotionally to their patients, even when the patient is a fellow physician. Even simple acknowledgments by our physicians of the incredible struggle we were enduring would have meant a lot to us.

My wife's illness and my experience as a family member changed the way I practiced medicine. As an epilepsy specialist, I had often asked my patients many questions. When did your seizures begin? What do your seizures look like? What anticonvulsants are you taking? Although I had always considered myself to be a sensitive physician, I now began to realize the importance of asking a completely different set of questions. What is it like for you to have seizures? Are you getting enough support at home? Are you very anxious about having seizures? Is there anything that we can do to help you cope with a difficult situation? I also wondered whether I had ever truly understood the difficulties experienced by many of my patients. In attempting to pay more attention to my patients' feelings, I instituted a policy in which patients awaiting entry into the office wrote down all the questions that they felt were important to discuss during their visits. I began to ask patients to complete a questionnaire that would alert me to possible anxiety or depression. I also intensified my working relationship with our local Epilepsy Foundation, designed protocols to assist patients with relaxation techniques, and helped out with support groups.

Very slowly but quite miraculously, my wife's illness began to recede. She regained consciousness, her paralysis resolved, and the chest tubes were removed. I like to think that if anything meaningful came out of this dreadful experience it was an enhanced empathy for my patients. I now devote much more of my time to writing and speaking at national symposia on topics that increase the awareness of health-care providers to the psychological needs of persons with epilepsy. When our offices are crammed with patients and distraught family members, when we face one emergency after another, when managed care organizations exert financial pressure on us, it is often difficult to keep the suffering of our patients in perspective. However, the most important lesson I have learned is how critical it is to interact with patients, not merely on the level of symptoms and medications but on a compassionate, humane level. Often, what is needed by the patient and family is not complicated; it involves moving away from the specifics of medical treatment to treating the whole person in the context of that patient's life experience.

So, now, the epileptologist who enters the intensive care unit to see a patient is not the same doctor he was before his wife became ill. Although I may not be as successful as I would like to be, I always try to express to my patients that I understand the ordeal they have been through.

I know that makes a difference. *The* difference.

42

We knew her phone number by heart. She called when she was injured or frightened, or just to talk. Her clinic visits were virtually all the same. She couldn't always recall the dosages of the medications she took.

The list of medications was extensive. Her husband, who accompanied her infrequently, orchestrated her medication regimen. It always amazed me that she could look so good in the office—animated and cheerful, makeup in place, and stylishly attired. The untrained observer would never suspect that she was coping with so many medical problems, including epilepsy.

Time and again, I was surprised that she had so little insight into her condition or her limitations. Nothing appeared to make her better. Most of the time, all that I could do was nod and listen to her frustration. I feared for her safety.

Each visit ended the same way. I would turn to leave the room and she would ask again, for the hundredth time, "Do you think these seizures will ever go away?"

I think she knows the answer, but I have to offer hope. Even for the hundredth time.

43

❖ ❖ ❖ ❖ ❖

Patients, residents, and students often ask me, "Why did you specialize in the treatment of patients with epilepsy?" I have a standard response about my long-standing interest in physiology and neurochemistry and how epilepsy combines these two sciences. Although that is often my professional response, I always think back to an episode that occurred over 25 years ago.

While in the junior high school lunchroom, my best friend suddenly cried out, stiffened, and fell backwards from his seat. He was jerking on the floor. At first we thought this was just typical lunchtime antics. As he was taken to the nurse's office, I realized it was much more than that. I remember listening with fascination to my friend's description of the neurologic examination he was given. I vividly recall his description of the test with the "wires and flashing lights" (the electroencephalogram). I listened without real understanding as he told me that he would be taking two medications for the rest of his life. His seizures were well controlled, and he went on to become very successful in his chosen profession.

Years later, while I was a neurology resident, my friend and I again lived in the same city. He was still taking two anticonvulsant medications. At my urging he switched neurologists and had his regimen simplified to a single medication. He continues to do well and recently married. I cannot help but believe that seeing my oldest and dearest friend have a seizure when we were in junior high school had some influence on my career choice.

Perhaps my answer to "Why epilepsy?" also has something to do with epilepsy itself. Because of the long-term nature of this disorder, I have been able to develop relationships with patients and their families that might not have been possible in other fields of medicine.

A resident once asked me, "Did you have any idea when *you* were a resident what was in store for you in the field of epilepsy?" I have learned over time that the correct answer is no. I never expected to be confronted by a teenaged boy and his mother saying, "Doctor, you are our last hope." This young man was not able to function because of his frequent complex partial seizures, which occurred day and night. Before our meeting, he had tried many medications and had almost died from a reaction to one of them. After he underwent a thorough evaluation, we decided that he should undergo a temporal lobectomy. He took our advice and was seizure-free for over a year. He decided to go off to college, where he continues today despite occasional nocturnal seizures. Seeing this person and others like him return to a normal life after all the hardships they have endured is what motivates me. Having this young man's father, with tears in his eyes, explain how he and his family truly appreciate my efforts is the icing on the cake!

44

There are two patients I will never forget.

J.W. was a 22-year-old woman when I first met her. Her seizures had begun at the age of 10. She had simple partial seizures, complex partial seizures, and rare generalized tonic–clonic seizures. Her seizures continued despite trials of many medications, and she was referred to me to see what I could do to improve her seizure control.

I learned that J.W. had a somewhat chaotic social history. She had completed high school but had never worked effectively. Recently, she had been emancipated from her family and was living independently in a hotel. Various charities actively helped her to maintain this existence. She had many hopes for her future, places she wanted to go and things she wanted to do.

J.W. had been followed fairly closely by the psychiatry service over the years and had taken various antidepressant and antipsychotic medications. Working with her was challenging; sometimes she was very argumentative, and at other times she could be very charming.

With intensive support from the epilepsy team, J.W. was able to go through with an inpatient evaluation for epilepsy surgery. The tests showed that her seizures came from her right mesial temporal region and that she had right mesial temporal sclerosis. Subsequently, she underwent a right temporal lobectomy.

That was several years ago. Because J.W. had no further seizures and complained about possible medication side effects—lack of libido and inability to achieve orgasm—she was gradually tapered off her seizure medication. She became gainfully employed, although her ability to stay in any one job was somewhat limited. She moved into a better residential environment.

J.W. became much more socially active and purchased a motorcycle, which was one of her deepest desires. She explored the state and the country on her motorcycle. However her social environment continued to be chaotic and her friends and acquaintances were frequently involved in altercations. She was hospitalized for depression several months ago and required electroshock therapy. This was difficult for her because she was afraid that the shock therapy might make her seizures come back.

After that admission, J.W. came into the seizure clinic, excited and hopeful about her long-term plans. She had a twinkle in her eye and a hearty laugh.

Recently, J.W. did achieve her fame, but certainly not her fortune. She was murdered, the first homicide in our city this year. Her lifestyle and poor judgment had led to her downfall: she had left a bar with the wrong person. The newspaper graphically described the discovery of her "nude, blood-smeared body" lying face down in the snow. The alleged murderer was apprehended, but the investigation and trial are yet to begin.

I will truly miss J.W. and her twinkle. I will miss seeing her gradually and slowly maturing and achieving her goals and aspirations. Perhaps her goals would not have been my goals for a young, fairly bright woman. But she had renewed hope and joy because she was seizure-free, was off medications, and could at last think of herself as a normal person. Remembering that gives me some comfort, as does knowing that I helped provide her with much-needed support.

T.W. was 19 years old when I first evaluated him for episodes of staring, confusion, strange repetitive movements, and occasional urinary incontinence. He had experienced these seizures up to four or five times a week, despite excellent compliance with medication trials and support from his family.

After graduating from high school, T.W. became employed. His special interests were etching and engraving, and he worked with glass and granite. He particularly missed not being able to drive, which hindered him from exploring other employment opportunities in his rural area.

T.W. persevered through further trials with medications, including investigational drugs. Although his seizures remained uncontrolled, he did not lose his sense of humor. Eventually he decided to find out if he was a candidate for epilepsy surgery. The evaluation showed that he was, and he underwent a right temporal lobectomy. Postoperatively, his cognitive abilities diminished mildly for a short period of time. He became seizure-free and tapered off his seizure medications.

T.W. has now been off medications for a year and remains seizure-free. He began his own business and works, in addition, for another employer. He has a car and drives. He even has a girlfriend. Occasionally he drinks a beer. He is actively involved with his family and his community and is incredibly pleased that he chose to "take the chance" with surgery.

I have seen T.W. develop from a somewhat shy and reticent young man into a productive member of his community. He is warm, considerate, and continues to have a sense of humor. He is looking forward to a fulfilling life.

Given this young man's ambition, his strength, and the support he receives from his family, I believe he will succeed.

45

I first experienced the excitement of attending the epilepsy clinic over 30 years ago. There has been no diminution in that sensation to this day.

I derive professional satisfaction from the first moment I see a patient through each follow-up visit. Epilepsy presents a variety of medical challenges that require an extensive understanding of neurophysiology, neuropathology, clinical pharmacology, and human behavior. The successful treatment of this complex disorder clearly requires competence in each of these areas. However, not all of this competence is derived from formal education. The cumulative insights that arise from following and treating patients provide a wealth of clinical experience that cannot be obtained from standard texts or other literature.

People with epilepsy suffer the consequences of prejudice, restricted education and transportation, and unemployment and underemployment, as well as many personal and family psychological traumas. These problems are often relatively easy for the physician to recognize but quite difficult to rectify because our training is inadequate in these areas. Assistance from other specialists is often required. This comprehensive approach to patient care is vital to achieve the best possible outcome.

Early in my career, I realized that each patient with seizures is unique and can teach us about a different facet of epilepsy. Applying that knowledge can sometimes be decidedly challenging, but those of us who help to resolve our patients' difficulties enjoy immense intellectual rewards. I also learned that epilepsy affects the patient's personality, feelings, and responses to others and to society. Clearly, physicians must comprehensively analyze these ongoing problems in the context of their patients' preexisting personalities and cognitive strengths. Even patients whose seizures do not substantially improve with medications may derive some comfort from simply discussing their problems and learning to deal with the consequences of their epilepsy.

I believe that both patients and their physicians should develop and maintain a long-term perspective on epilepsy and drug therapy. Personal and medical crises arise from time to time, but life is a continuum regardless of the eruptions and disruptions caused by seizures and medications. Whether or not epilepsy becomes the major theme for a person or his/her family or remains only a ripple in that continuum bears greatly on the person's subsequent enjoyment of life. Patients who become consumed with their epilepsy appear to have the most difficulty in achieving a fulfilling life. Seizure control should not be all-important—there is too much more to life.

I believe that these points are illustrated by J.B., a patient of mine for the past 22 years. She began having nocturnal tonic–clonic seizures when she was 19 years old, 1 month after the delivery of her first child. I first saw her when she was 23. She had been hospitalized for seizures described as air hunger, nervousness, left arm numbness, dimming of vision, lightheadedness, and the perception of a peculiar bad odor. She would then collapse to the floor, unable to respond but still aware of her environment. The referring neurologist had obtained an EEG and, because it was normal, concluded that her seizures were psychogenic, especially considering their unusual character and her recent depression.

J.B. was a pretty, slightly plump, ingratiating young woman with mild facial freckling. A slight twang was noticeable in her otherwise pleasant southern drawl. Initially there was some unsteadiness when she walked, but this cleared within a day. Neuropsychological testing found verbal memory impairment and tendencies toward hysteria and attention-seeking behavior. Her computed axial tomography scan and pneumoencephalogram were normal. Application of special EEG leads and induction of prolonged sleep revealed a spike and slow-wave focus from the left temporal lobe.

I believed that J.B. had epilepsy. The new EEG information and the history of nocturnal seizures strongly suggested the diagnosis of left temporal lobe epilepsy, characterized by complex partial seizures and secondarily generalized tonic–clonic seizures. Although I concurred that she might also have pseudoseizures, simply because she had a somewhat hysterical personality did not mean that *all* her behavior, including seizures, was emotionally derived. Still, it was difficult to sort out the interaction of epilepsy and her personality, the influence of medications on her behavior, and how to reconcile her symptoms with her actual seizure frequency.

I realized that it made little difference whether some of J.B.'s events were not seizures, except when it came to determining how often her epileptic seizures were occurring—but that would remain my problem.

J.B. required treatment for seizures as well as psychological support, particularly to help her function as a housewife and mother with epilepsy. These other needs were addressed by involving key members of our comprehensive epilepsy team—the social worker, epilepsy nurse, and rehabilitation counselor—in her care. Their input would prove to be of substantial long-term benefit in helping her to deal with seizures, to cope with many other issues at home, and to analyze her educational and vocational prospects for the future.

After being discharged from the hospital, J.B. continued to have several seizures each day. During some of the seizures she felt weak, lay down, and then folded her arms, grasped her upper arms, and had rhythmic jerks of her arms and head. When these seizures became more frequent, J.B.'s mother left her job as a nurse so that she could help J.B. take care of her children. At her mother's urging, J.B. and her family moved into a trailer in the mother's yard.

Under my supervision, J.B. underwent an evaluation for epilepsy surgery. The tests revealed that her seizures began in the left temporal lobe. Plans for surgery were abandoned, however, when the neuropsychologist interpreted the intracarotid amobarbital test as showing that J.B. had difficulty with memory function in the right hemisphere. I was frustrated by the amobarbital test results. I am afraid that I let my guard down and let her see my disappointment. She did not need to be burdened with my frustration; her problems far outweighed mine.

The next year I saw J.B. for another type of seizure, during which she banged her head with her fists. On one occasion I found her stretched out in a wheelchair and hyperventilating. Her eyes closed quickly when I tried to open them. Her pupils were reactive, and her neurologic exam and blood pressure were normal. She improved promptly after breathing into a paper bag. I then learned that she was under psychological stress, having witnessed a train wreck in which two people were killed. However, I further discovered that the level of one of her seizure drugs was in the toxic range. Adjusting the dose stopped this new type of psychogenic seizure, teaching me once again that antiepileptic drug therapy may affect behavior in unusual ways.

I left for a sabbatical and did not see J.B. for over 4 years. By that time her typical seizures were refractory to medical treatment. Her husband was so willing to see her proceed with another surgical evaluation that he was prepared to pay for it out of pocket. Reevaluation at our epilepsy center again demonstrated the left temporal lobe epileptic focus. This time, though, the sodium amobarbital study was interpreted differently. J.B. indeed had reasonably good memory function in the right hemisphere. I was delighted, and felt that we could finally proceed with surgery. Unfortunately, her husband was severely injured in a fall and fractured his back, so her surgery again had to wait.

Eventually, J.B. successfully underwent a left temporal lobectomy. Unbeknownst to me, the surgeon had arranged for her to be admitted to the university hospital as a teaching case. Consequently, the university absorbed all the costs of her surgery.

J.B. returned to see me 3 months after surgery and reported that she had experienced a 30-second "sinking spell" at a television studio just before a live interview about her medical experiences and success with epilepsy surgery. She recovered quickly and did a great job. That was her last seizure.

At our last visit about a year ago, J.B. was outgoing, self-assured, and pleased with her accomplishments. She told me about her activities and the things that she planned to do. She spoke often on behalf of the local epilepsy association. She talked with other potential surgical candidates and shared her experiences. She helped to take care of her grandchildren.

To this day I am proud of J.B., not because of what I contributed to her care but because of what she has been able to endure—the many ups and downs, frequent hardships, and imposed limitations—and because of what she has had the strength to accomplish. She has been able to achieve a great degree of fulfillment and satisfaction in her life. Despite her years-long ordeal with epilepsy, she never permitted it to become the primary focus of her life. She may have required and accepted assistance from time to time, but with this help she successfully raised two children and maintained a positive relationship with her husband.

I have learned several important lessons from J.B. First, diagnostic tests are not infallible. A review of the circumstances surrounding the first amobarbital test eventually led me to challenge the conclusion and repeat the test. Perhaps I should have done this earlier, but there were extenuating circumstances. Second, medical and surgical treatments are not perfect. Third, both patient and doctor must be tolerant, persistent, and methodical to optimize therapy. Finally, persistent medical assessment and reassessment may be required to achieve success in treating epilepsy. It is important, as amply demonstrated by this story, that personality characteristics are allowed to cloud the diagnostic issues. From the very beginning, J.B. and I both held out hope that eventually we could resolve her difficulties with epilepsy. And we did.

Yes, I am still excited when I attend the epilepsy clinic.

46

To say that I was uneducated about epilepsy before working in an epilepsy clinic is an understatement. My only previous exposure had been an incident that had occurred when I was a teenager: I had witnessed my brother-in-law having a grand mal seizure. I remember my mother forcing the back of a spoon into his mouth to "stop him from swallowing his tongue."

My education began with my first project: entering information about epilepsy into a computer from slides that were used to educate health-care professionals about the many different aspects of epilepsy. It turned out that there couldn't have been a better introduction to the world of epilepsy and the effect of this disorder on those with seizures and on their families and friends.

This work was enlightening but somewhat technical and did not evoke any significant feelings toward the patients. It was, however, a shock to learn that there was more to epilepsy than grand mal seizures.

To further my knowledge of epilepsy, I decided to read a book that contained stories written by people with epilepsy—the first book in the *Brainstorms* series. I remember that night clearly. My husband and children were asleep, and I was alone in our family room. I recall that I managed to read only a few of the stories before I was forced to put the book down, because a feeling of absolute horror completely overwhelmed me. I could not imagine going through life having to deal with the difficulties that most of the people in the book seemed to just accept. I could not fathom what it would be like knowing that every time I felt happy, I could expect to have a seizure. Or going out to a restaurant knowing that at any time I could have a seizure and remove my clothes.

My first instinct was not to finish reading the book. I set it aside and tried to ignore it, but finally I forced myself to continue. It took three evenings to read, during which time I found myself having some of the symptoms described in the book. I found myself questioning whether certain things that had happened to me in the past could have been seizures. But most of all, while reading this book I felt awed by and admiration for most of the writers, who had managed to deal with all the problems epilepsy had brought their way and to do so with dignity and perseverance. As time passed and I began meeting some of the same people whose lives I had read about, I discovered that I felt sympathy for them but never pity.

Now, during the course of a single week at the clinic, I can experience any number of different feelings. Disappointment when a patient who has been seizure-free for a period of time has a seizure; absolute joy when another patient is finally seizure-free after years of medication changes, side effects, and sometimes surgery. Anger when someone uses epilepsy as an excuse to manipulate and control those around him or blames the disorder for whatever ills may happen to befall him, whether or not they are related to epilepsy. Compassion for parents whose child has just received a diagnosis of epilepsy. Frustration for the young person who has to travel such a harsh and difficult road.

And, for me, the most difficult feeling to deal with is the utter helplessness I feel when a patient with whom I am speaking on the phone suddenly has a seizure. I can hear the patient, but there is nothing I can do except stay on the line until the seizure passes and I can assure myself that the person is okay. When a patient has a seizure in the clinic, the feeling of helplessness is not as strong because there is at least something to be done—making sure the patient is safe and will not get hurt during the seizure or calling for help if a doctor or nurse is not present. Not much in the big scheme of things but something proactive nevertheless.

Working on a daily basis with persons who have epilepsy has colored my life to a certain extent, mostly for the better. On the negative side, I tend to worry more about my two teenagers being hurt doing the usual things teenagers do, like riding bikes, playing sports, and driving. It is my greatest fear and one that I try not to dwell on. It almost feels as though I shouldn't even be writing about it! On the positive side, there is never a dull moment during my day as the trials, tribulations, and successes of the patients become mine. The most rewarding part of this job is interacting with some wonderful, interesting people who have learned to use humor and courage to handle the blows life has dealt them.

I can say with all honesty that I love my job and all the ups and downs that go along with it. The personal relationships I have developed with many patients with intractable epilepsy more than make up for the times when I could cheerfully strangle a particularly demanding person whose seizures are few and side effects nonexistent.

It is truly a privilege to work with the patients, nurses, physicians, and support staff that make up this epilepsy clinic of ours.

47

My first experience with epilepsy occurred when I was a child. I was 7 years old, my brother Jerry was 5, and my brother John was 2. My mother was taking us with her to pick up my father from work because his car was in the shop. Unbeknownst to my mother, John had a fever. He didn't appear to be sick.

We three boys were sitting in the back seat of the station wagon. Suddenly, I noticed that something was happening to 2-year-old John. His body stiffened and then began to shake, so I called to my mother that something was wrong. She pulled the car over and then laid my brother down on the back seat. He was still convulsing. My 5-year-old brother Jerry and I were already frightened. Then my mother, obviously distraught, turned to some people who were walking on the sidewalk and cried, "Please help me! My baby's having a convulsion!" My mother was a former operating room nurse and I had never seen her lose her cool in an emergency. Jerry and I began to cry uncontrollably. My mother saw how frightened we were and then told us to say some prayers for John. I know I have never since prayed as hard as I did that day.

We brought John to the pediatrician, who wasn't very far away. It turned out that John had had a simple febrile seizure. He never had another one, and his development after the seizure was normal.

As a neurologist, I often hear family members in my office describe how scary it is to watch their loved one have a tonic–clonic seizure.

I'll always know how they feel.

48

As a psychotherapist and a group leader for an epilepsy support group, I am struck by the enormous burden that the diagnosis of epilepsy imposes on patients and their families.

I am reminded of one woman who joined my support group after seizures developed during menopause. At her first session, she said that when the doctor told her she had seizures, she declared, "Thank God it's not epilepsy!" Since then, she has been struggling with the diagnosis of epilepsy and has had to totally rearrange her life. She has faced job discrimination and a number of losses. She is not able to drive. As a grandmother, she finds herself in a reversed role—she is the one being taken care of now.

To help herself cope with the enormous impact of the diagnosis, she entered into a therapeutic relationship with me. Now, 3 years later, she is doing significantly better with both seizure control and managing her life. She is working at a job that makes her feel validated and has become an advocate for herself and others.

Another woman, who received the diagnosis of epilepsy at age 15, was told that she needed brain surgery to alleviate her seizures. At that time she was a young mother of a 3-year-old boy and decided to wait to undergo the surgery until he was no longer a baby. The operation was only marginally successful because she continued to have grand mal seizures and was admitted to the hospital on a near-monthly basis in status epilepticus.

When the woman first came to my group, she was tearful and depressed. She wondered if she would ever be able to function again without the daily fear of a seizure tearing her away from her family and herself. In the group, she learned that she was not alone with her epilepsy and that others struggled with the same disorder. She began to keep fastidious records of her seizure activity—for example, when she took medication, exercised, or ate. Faithfully, she and her spouse recorded her seizures. They began to notice a pattern. She was greatly relieved to note that her seizures occurred with some regularity around the time of her ovulation and that she could predict when she was most vulnerable to having them. This realization empowered her. She was able to modify her lifestyle so that she could ride out the storm rather than have it control her. Now she is experiencing far fewer seizures and works part time, something she never believed would be possible.

These two people embody the great fortitude that I have observed in people who suffer from epilepsy. They have a great appreciation for the little things in life that most of us take for granted, such as being aware of what we have said, to whom, and in what manner.

When a seizure occurs after a long seizure-free period, both the patient and the caregiver may feel helpless. It is then terribly painful to sit and listen to the patient wonder what he or she did wrong to bring on the seizure. Self-blame and self-torture, shame, and anger are powerful emotions felt by patients that must be acknowledged and managed.

As a therapist, I am challenged by patients who worry every day that a seizure will send them back to square one, forcing them to rebuild everything that they had gained. Sometimes the cyclical nature of epilepsy makes working with such people like a revolving door. No sooner are you through the entrance on your way to your destination than you are whisked out to start all over again.

49

To the neuroscientist in me, caring for patients with epilepsy is fascinating. I never tire of hearing people describe the thoughts and feelings that they experience during a seizure. It is a great challenge to try to sort through their descriptions of strange sensations, bizarre behavior, and the like, and to combine that with the neurologic examination and arrive at a diagnosis. It is gratifying to be able to explain a patient's "spells" that have defied diagnosis for a long time.

Like most people, I strongly identify with the famous axiom of Descartes, "I think therefore I am"*(Discours de la Methode*, 1637). That is why, in my view, the most striking consequences of seizures are the loss of a patient's ability to think, to maintain awareness, and to control his or her actions.

The unpredictability of this loss of control, and the associated fear, hover over most people with epilepsy, giving them a vague, ever-present sense of unease and isolation. The alienation that patients feel is further magnified when they are excluded from the daily activities, such as driving, that the rest of us take for granted. It also profoundly shakes their self-identity and self-confidence.

It is not surprising that patients with epilepsy, given these burdens, express a great deal of heartache and depression in the doctor's office. More often than not, somebody with epilepsy cries during the course of one of my 4-hour clinic sessions.

Another feeling expressed by patients is guilt. Because we believe inherently in the idea of causality, that everything happens for a specific reason, we are psychologically troubled when we cannot find a good explanation for events that occur around us. For so many people with epilepsy, no clear reason for their seizures has been found. This makes them angry, which I can understand. But I was surprised to find that so many people also feel guilty—in particular, guilty about some previous errant act that they are convinced is the original cause of their epilepsy.

The sense of guilt may be more intense when the cause of epilepsy is actually known, especially for parents who have a child with seizures. When parents bring an adult child with epilepsy to see me for yet another clinic visit, they occasionally allude to their long-vanished hopes of raising their child to become an accomplished adult. They often recall an incident some 20, 30, or 40 years earlier when their baby squirmed off a table, fell off a bike, ran into the street chasing a ball, or suffered some other tragedy in an unattended moment. In an instant, all their hopes and dreams for their child were shattered. Years later, they continue to feel guilty about their responsibility for that incident and additional guilt for what they imagine will happen to their child after they die. As a parent blessed with healthy, bright children, I can only imagine how these parents must feel.

Caring for patients with epilepsy is a privilege. I feel a sense of anger or even outrage when patients describe the shoddy and, at times, flagrantly incompetent treatment they have received from previous health-care providers. Perhaps this is because I believe that being a physician is a special calling that is afforded to only a select few. Physicians are given glimpses of the most precious and intimate thoughts and feelings of their patients.

The daily challenge before me is to make sure that I take care of each patient with epilepsy in a manner that is worthy of this special responsibility.

50

In discussing the psychosocial implications of seizures, people usually consider only generalized convulsions or complex partial seizures. But I have learned that patients with more subtle seizures may be equally affected by epilepsy.

I once cared for a patient, an accountant, who had only simple partial seizures. His seizures occurred several times a week and affected his performance at work because his concentration was impaired from the seizures. We enrolled him in a research antiepileptic drug protocol.

Fortunately, he became seizure-free during the research study. His performance at work greatly improved, and his tennis game (his favorite pastime) benefited from improved hand–eye coordination. But then reports of several deaths among patients taking this antiepileptic drug led the manufacturer to recommend discontinuing its use in patients whose quality of life had not drastically improved. My patient was counseled and told about the risks of continuing to take the medication. He felt that the benefit outweighed the risk because he was more alert and had dramatic improvement in his quality of life. This patient continues to take this medication and remains seizure-free.

After my involvement in the care of this patient, I learned that it does not matter what type of seizure a patient has or how often these seizures occur. All types of seizures are devastating to some patients, whether or not they interfere with consciousness or happen once a day, once a month, or once a year. What is more important is the *patient's* perspective. How the patient perceives epilepsy in the context of his or her life must be understood and acknowledged by the patient's care providers and integrated into the treatment plan.

51

❖ ❖ ❖ ❖ ❖

When I started out as a neurologist, my scientific and medical training had me well prepared to provide medical treatment for patients with epilepsy. I initially regarded epilepsy as strictly a medical condition that could be well controlled with antiepileptic drugs in the majority of patients. I had little knowledge about the psychosocial consequences of epilepsy, nor did I see any reason to acquire such knowledge.

I quickly learned that the psychosocial aspects were sometimes much more important than just controlling seizures. I also learned that modern medical techniques may not be sufficient to prevent some of the serious and devastating consequences of epilepsy.

Over many years of treating hundreds of people with epilepsy, I have been emotionally touched by the personal misfortunes of some of my patients and I have learned to appreciate that epilepsy may be a very malignant disorder on a personal level. The patient I describe here has taught me that sometimes what we offer our patients in terms of compassion, friendship, and understanding makes a bigger difference in their lives than our medical treatment.

Mary is a 28-year-old patient whom I met 12 years ago. She had a history of primary generalized epilepsy with absence, atonic, and tonic–clonic seizures poorly controlled on multiple antiepileptic drugs. Over the next several years I prescribed a number of different medication regimens, trying to convert her to monotherapy. These attempts were unsuccessful, and she continued to have frequent, predominantly atonic seizures.

Mary subsequently became pregnant. Ultrasound examinations during early pregnancy were negative and alpha-fetoprotein plasma levels were normal. We were both reassured, because we knew that the fetus would be considered at high risk for birth defects from Mary's uncontrolled seizures and multiple medications.

Contrary to what these modern diagnostic techniques had indicated, Mary subsequently delivered at 39 weeks, by cesarean section, a female infant with a large lumbosacral meningomyelocele, a moderate-sized ventricular septal defect, talipes equinovarus, severe leg contractures, hirsutism, a flattened nasal ridge, hypertelorism, and a wide maxilla.

The father did not accept the child. He disappeared, unable to provide any support at the time it was most needed. Mary was unable to provide proper care for her child, who was placed in the care of a health agency.

Mary has continued to have seizures, despite undergoing a partial and then total corpus callosotomy. She continues on polytherapy. Trials of the new antiepileptic drugs have not been successful.

Mary has benefited very little from our armamentarium of epilepsy treatments, and she has paid a great price for her epilepsy. I continue to look after Mary, and I can only hope that my support and compassion comfort her. I feel that Mary has made me a better physician by making me realize the importance of caring for the patient as a *person* and not just as a *medical disorder*, particularly when our antiepileptic drugs fail to improve seizure control.

Mary reminds us of the dictum "primum non nocere." First, do no harm.

52

I have been a clinical epileptologist for four decades, since the end of World War II. At that time, it was common for medical students to work as research assistants for both pocket money and experience.

I was assigned to work in an endocrinology laboratory that was engaged in the study of calcium metabolism. This research drew me to the central nervous system, but I was much more impressed by the sister of a fellow student in the laboratory due to her epilepsy. She had been born in the Dutch East Indies and had suffered from cerebral malaria as a child. She had done very well in school until she was 11 years old, when she developed complex partial seizures.

After an intellectually challenging period of neurological study at the Salpetriere in Paris, I decided to become a neurologist and then to pursue my interest in epilepsy. My neurology residency, however, soon made it clear to me that an urge to heal is not a desirable asset for anyone wishing to pursue neurology unless he or she is prepared for extreme frustration. But I also found that epilepsy was the exception—among the neurological disorders, epilepsy was one of the few disorders for which interventions were better than simple letting nature run its course.

Early in my career, I became concerned about the therapeutic environment in which patients with chronic disorders such as epilepsy were treated. University hospitals were not the most suitable place—the rapid turnover of physicians, all of whom try to become fully informed about the patient's history, forces patients to rehash their medical history again and again. This situation makes patients feel that no real progress is being made. How much better it would be, I thought, for patients with epilepsy to be cared for by one specialist over many years, so that both the patients and the doctor could experience the ups and downs of the patients' condition over time. In fact, the movement toward establishing this type of care environment had already begun. In the later 19th century, a German Protestant minister founded an epilepsy center in Bielefeld, Germany, which he named Bethel. This center became a model for similar institutions in Europe and the United States and was the inspiration for the establishment of the Dutch epilepsy center in which I worked for several decades until my retirement.

At our epilepsy center, I was involved in the day-to-day care of several hundred people. Now as I contemplate my past experiences, many anecdotal stories come to mind. There are the sad stories of patients whose seizures were symptomatic of inoperable tumors. In those cases, there were often long periods of relative stability during which patients and families needed to be supported while the sword of Damocles swung over their heads. Devastating, rapid decline and death inevitably followed these periods with families left behind in disarray.

Then I think of young children in whom epilepsy was recognized but not further characterized as a syndrome—in those cases, I could provide a miracle cure by simply diagnosing the epilepsy syndrome and selecting appropriate treatment.

Unlike epilepsy specialists elsewhere, we made house calls. I found these home visits to be particularly revealing. It is much easier to understand the anxiety of the family about their loved one suffering a major motor or complex partial seizure when you see that they live in a small apartment with cheap glass-topped tables and a bedroom so tiny that to fall between the bed and the wall during a seizure would be disastrous.

Why have I worked in the field of epilepsy for 40 years? There are three reasons: the people with epilepsy who I have treated, the progress that has been achieved in the understanding of seizures, and because of my colleagues around the world.

53

They would always come together to the clinic, mother and son. He was slightly built, in his early forties, and had started to lose his hair. Despite many efforts over the years, his partial epilepsy with rare tonic–clonic seizures remained uncontrollable. In addition, he suffered from a mild cognitive disability that nevertheless allowed him to work in a sheltered workshop during the day. Each evening he would return home to his mother. His mother was a tall, very strong-willed person in her late seventies who had brought up her son by herself.

When it became clear that treatment could not cure her son's epilepsy, our talks in the clinic centered more and more on the need for him to become less dependent and to begin to live his own life. Easier said than done, especially because his mother constantly worried about seizure-related accidents despite my reassurances that a serious accident was unlikely if he avoided swimming, which he never did anyway. When I learned that the son was considering taking a week-long trip together with his buddies at the workshop, I encouraged him to join them and eventually convinced his anxious mother to let him go.

You can therefore imagine my horror and sense of guilt when the mother called a few days later to tell me that her son had suddenly died while on the outing with his friends. "My son was said by the other fellows to have had one of his seizures, which they knew about. He fell down and hurt his head, but he got up after a while and joined the others. Several hours later he felt drowsy and was told by the supervisor to retire early. The next morning he was found dead in bed."

A few weeks later, the mother called for an appointment. For the first time she came into my office without her son, dressed in black.

I expected her to blame me indirectly for the death of her son, because I had encouraged him to go. To my great relief, she said nothing of the sort. "I do miss my son and hope he did not suffer. I am glad it is over for him. But I have to tell you that I am also relieved at the same time. You know, my greatest fear was that I might die before my son and leave him all alone. His death saved me from that horror."

54

Working as a pediatric therapist with brain-injured children is sometimes agonizing but, at other times, gratifying. Many of my students suffer from seizure disorders and from the many side effects of anticonvulsant medications. As a professional, I feel most useful when I can offer support and encouragement by means of hugs and education to exhausted parents and their exceptional children. The endless visits to neurologists and therapists have caused these families to lose a great deal of time and various aspects of normal development.

One particular morning will always burn in my memory. Before class, I listened to a distraught teacher lament over her son's decision to change his college major from premed to liberal arts. Several hours later, one of my students, Jimmy, went into a blank stare, and then a major convulsion. For what seemed like an eternity, he thrashed around and made strange noises. When the seizure was over, Jimmy was gasping for air and briefly became unconscious.

Some very intense emotions occur after a seizure, even for caregivers. Once more, I had to face a duty that I dreaded—calling Jimmy's mom. I heard her sigh over the phone with sad resignation. I remembered our last conversation, when she had talked about the financial toll of taking off time from work, the emotional roller coaster of having a sick child, and the feelings of helplessness she had.

Jimmy's mom soon arrived to take her sleeping child home to recover. She wrapped him in a blanket with heartbreaking tenderness and fatigue. The years of living with his seizures were etched on her face.

As I hugged her good-bye, I wondered what was so bad about liberal arts.

55

Epilepsy holds a special place among neurologic disorders. Not only is it one of the more eminently treatable of these disorders but it appears to be fundamentally different from other brain problems. Whereas much of neurology deals with the treatment of disorders characterized by a persistent loss of function, epilepsy represents the entire gamut of brain function. Episodes of excessive brain activity are often followed by transient brain dysfunction. Except for the rather obvious example of generalized convulsions, the diversity of clinical presentations often renders the diagnosis of epilepsy difficult. During my training I had the opportunity to treat epilepsy in a patient whose condition demonstrated to me the uniqueness of epilepsy patients and the empirical nature of their treatment.

A middle-aged man, who worked as a truck driver, began having spells in which he would experience an unusual, nauseated feeling in his upper abdomen and then lose consciousness. His wife related that he would fall to the ground, become rigid, and have a brief convulsion, after which he would regain consciousness fairly rapidly. His primary care physician prescribed one and then two antiepileptic medications for him, but without success. The patient was sent to a pulmonary specialist, who told him that he should return to work. He was ultimately referred to me for a neurologic evaluation. I concluded from my evaluation that I had insufficient data to diagnose his condition accurately, and the man was admitted to the hospital for inpatient video/EEG monitoring.

While the patient's medications were being tapered, he experienced two partial seizures. With each seizure his heart rate rapidly decreased and his cardiac ventricular contractions ceased. Within 10 seconds his brain activity, as measured by the EEG, slowed and disappeared. He became rigid, had two to three clonic jerks, and rapidly regained awareness after his heart function had returned to normal. In short, every time he had a seizure, his heart would stop, and the resulting convulsive syncope or fainting spell would abort the seizure.

I was particularly fascinated by this patient because he was experiencing two diametrically opposed brain events. The relative absence of brain activity during his syncope was incompatible with the excessively rhythmic activity of the seizure. So, in a sense, he had a built-in mechanism of seizure cessation. Feeling rather full of myself, I presented the diagnosis to him in a self-congratulatory manner and consulted a cardiologist. For fear that the patient's heart would not restart after one of his seizures, we decided that he should have a pacemaker placed, and this procedure was done.

Soon thereafter, it became apparent that we had removed this man's intrinsic safety mechanism against seizures and he began to experience secondarily generalized tonic–clonic seizures because his seizures were no longer aborted by cessation of cardiac—and then cortical—function. His seizures ultimately proved refractory to other antiepileptic medications. Because he could no longer drive, an application for disability benefits was made but denied. In the stressful months that followed, he began to experience unusual events in addition to his typical seizures. These new episodes were ultimately determined to be psychogenic.

I have long since left training, but I continue to remember that particular patient. Although I believe that pacemaker placement was an appropriate measure in his case, I question whether I had a beneficial effect on the man's life. In many ways, his story highlights the contrast between the diagnostic power produced by knowledge of epilepsy and the weakness that accompanies the inability to treat seizures adequately in a patient whose disorder we believe we understand. For me, that patient serves as a reminder that although we strive to make neurology a science, it remains a largely empirical pursuit.

The challenge of clinical epileptology is in the judicious and individualized application of a few accepted principles of treatment to a specific patient. Through research, the insights gained by use of these principles will continue to increase, but individualization of treatment will remain the cornerstone of treating patients with epilepsy for many years to come.

56

I was frightened as a child when I watched my father in status epilepticus. I used to say the same prayer every day. Please, God, let my father be free of seizures.

My father was 35 years old when he had his first seizure caused by cysticercosis. He was the father of five children. A professor of medicinal chemistry, he was a brilliant young man with a promising future, the youngest faculty member to become a professor at his university.

I watched my father deteriorate over the years, having one seizure after another, until I could no longer recognize him. Because he took anticonvulsants his seizures were infrequent, but those he had almost always progressed to status epilepticus. My mother used to have my uncles carry him while she ran out to the street like a mad woman, crying out for a taxi. By the time they arrived at the nearest hospital, 3 to 4 hours later, my father had stopped having seizures and nothing more could be done. My mother's elders told her that the best thing she could do for her husband when he was having a seizure was to cover him with a blanket, clear out the room, and let the seizure run its course. After many frantic and futile runs to the hospital, my mother became convinced of the elders' collective wisdom and let my father's seizures come and go and pass on their own. One day, he had one seizure after another, all day long. After that, he lost his job, his memory, and his intelligence. My father eventually lost his life to seizures.

I was the only girl in my family and my father's favorite child. Before he became so ill, we took many evening walks, holding hands. With my little fingers gently enclosed in his big hand, he would whisper to me, "What will my little girl be when she grows up?"

He would be proud to know that I grew up to become an epileptologist. I want to help patients and their families by being a partner in their lifelong struggle with epilepsy. I *feel* their pain, their fear, and their sadness, for they are mine as well.

57

We did not realize at first that the boy's illness was progressive. It came on seemingly out of nowhere and began slowly unraveling his adolescent life. His EEG was startlingly abnormal, and the jerks that began to occur with his every movement were interfering with his eating and other daily activities. He himself was mildly amused by the jerks, watching his hand and arm jump as he tried to put his Walkman on. I guess he thought of them as only a nuisance, maybe because he figured that we would fix the jerking with our complex drug regimens and the big, scary pills in odd shapes and colors.

Within days, though, we knew that the boy had an inherited disease that would become progressively worse and would essentially remain beyond the touch of the healing magic wand of science. Nature had outwitted us again, right before our eyes, claiming a very young one of us for its own special, deviant purpose.

The holidays were approaching, and I was much more used to caring for adults than kids. I still needed more emotional armor or a system of rationalization—or something—to cope easily with caring for such a young and ill patient, especially at Christmas time. Of course, I kept thinking of my child at home. And the boy's family situation was not the best; it was a family like many others, with its own complex interplay of divorce and step-parents, siblings, and half-siblings; and passion for alcohol. The family needed to gather their strength and obtain some hands-on help to cope with this new problem. They wanted us to help him and we would try.

We adjusted the boy's medications and started a new one, which caused the drop seizures and convulsions to improve quite a bit, but the jerks were still there. Even the EEG got better. I was trying to arrange for all of his tests and consultations to be completed soon enough for him to go home by Christmas, but this turned out to be impossible. He was shocked, then angry, then tearful. I reassured him that his family would come and bring him his presents and that special holiday meals and services would be available in the hospital. He blamed me for everything. He cried and cried and twisted my heart.

For the next few days, when I made rounds, the boy would usually ignore me. Amazingly, I found myself doing the only thing I could do for him then—feeding him. I felt that I was almost robotically fulfilling my role as a person who helps others as well as I can, with both doctor and patient facing a devastating situation. He needed to eat but couldn't open the packages of hospital food, put dressing on his salad, or spoon the soup into his mouth. I did these things for him, and he let me feed him, both of us feeling better that something positive was accomplished.

On Christmas Day the boy's brother visited him, bearing gifts. My patient demanded to go home and relentlessly questioned me, his unhappiness escalating. He intermittently asked for his mother. Finally he worked himself into a wordless, tearful state, and I knew that he was trying to communicate something more about his unhappiness, something more than just going home would resolve. Even the little brother was trying to console his inexplicably twitching big brother. I pushed my patient to talk and tell me more, and then it burst out.

"I don't care about the presents! I don't care if it's Christmas! I want to go home! I'm scared here. I've never been in a hospital before. I've never been sick!" the boy sputtered in a shaky, blurry New York accent. I realized that he was merely stating the obvious: he was young, very sick, and very scared. Going home would at least provide the relief of a familiar, if slightly chaotic, environment. My heart was ripped apart and I couldn't leave the room until he settled down, which wasn't until his mother came. Of course, I maintained my calm, clinical demeanor, but inside I felt as though I personally wanted to do battle with the messed-up strands of DNA that made the boy so sick and so unhappy, if they would only reveal themselves to me.

Most of the time I can help my patients do better by means of a combination of medications or surgery, lifestyle changes, or subtle attitude adjustments. I can also refer them to social services that provide routes to greater life fulfillment. But this time all I could do was listen carefully to my patient and feed him when he couldn't do it for himself.

It is not easy to look on the countenance of illness, for sometimes it mercilessly stares back.

58

I'll never forget the first time I met Julie. I was a first-year neurology resident, getting a pretty rough-and-tumble introduction to our "Friday outpatient mentored experience"—that is, residents' clinic. I walked through the lobby in my fine starched white coat and asked Amanda, the receptionist, where my next patient was. She pointed to the far corner of the waiting room to a heavy-set young woman who was asleep and snoring loudly. Amanda, who knew all the patients at least as well as we residents did, told me that Julie had been coming here to the Neurology Clinic for over 20 years. "She had some kind of childhood brain infection that gave her really bad seizures," Amanda added. Amanda had witnessed them many times in the waiting room—the blank stare, the chewing movements, the eye blinking, and then the terrible generalized convulsions that followed. Luckily, Julie rarely hurt herself during a seizure. Each time she had seen Julie seize, Amanda had asked her if she wanted to go the emergency room. Julie would just look up at her and smile with a kind of dazed look and say, "No, thank you, I'm not sure they would see me anyhow because I'm still paying off the $10,000 I owe them. At $10 a month I should be straight in about 400 years if all goes well." She would then giggle and say that unfortunately my hospital was next in line to be paid after two other hospitals and a few other emergency rooms on her side of town.

I walked quietly over to the corner and sat down next to the sleeping woman. Her intermittent snores were loud and there were occasional long, worrisome spaces between some of her breaths. After a moment or two she stirred, looked me square in the eyes, and said, "You're Dr. Witt, aren't ya?" I said, "Yes, how did you know?" Julie replied, "Each year when my senior resident gets ready to leave, I ask him who he recommends for my next doctor. I make a couple of phone calls and then decide on one of them. You're it."

With that brief introduction, we walked back to the examining room, both of us knowing full well who was in charge—her. On the way I asked Julie whether she always snored loudly and felt tired during the day. She replied, "Only when I take the bus." Bus apnea, bus apnea, I thought to myself. This was one neurological disorder that I had missed hearing about during my training. "What do you mean?" I asked. She answered, "Well, because my seizures are so bad I don't drive, so in order to get to the clinic here from across town, I have to get up at 4:30 in the morning to catch the bus." I looked at my watch. It was a quarter past 10:00. "What time did you get here?" I asked her. "Oh, about 7:30. The bus transfers take at least 3 hours. I usually find someone to let me into the building and then I try to take a nap before my office visit. It helps me stay awake when I talk to the doctor, particularly when I'm taking all this medicine."

I looked through Julie's three thick volumes of hospital charts, noting that she had been hospitalized at age 3 or 4 with severe seizures and a presumed brain infection. The seizures had come mercilessly ever since. Julie had undergone electroencephalography periodically throughout her childhood, but the patterns were unclear and no firm diagnosis was ever made. Generalized, focal, multifocal seizures—the chart was full of interpretations, none of which seemed to have helped her very much. She had tried practically every medication I knew plus a few I didn't. Admittedly, at that point in my training I did not know very much about epilepsy, but I knew this patient was going to be a challenging problem.

I continued on and asked, "Do you have a seizure calendar?" She said, "Sure," and fished some rumpled papers out of her purse. That calendar was one of the most impressive records of bravery I have ever seen. Some of the entries were as follows: "July 5: went to work. Still on probation. Had a seizure while stocking the salad bar. Spilled five gallons of russian dressing all over the floor. Woke up with the ambulance crew there, a bruise on my knee, and covered with russian dressing. God, I hate dressing." The next entry three days later read, "Woke up in the local emergency room. Bump on my head. Remember running to catch the bus and that's all." The calendar went on and on. Julie was having generalized convulsive seizures approximately two to three times a week. There were other, briefer events as well. "My boss at the Holiday Hotel found me in the kitchen, staring, with two of my fingers in boiling soup. Said he wondered why I didn't seem to feel any pain. Helped me bandage my fingers before he fired me." I noticed a scar on the back of Julie's left hand and asked about it. "That's from my last job," she replied, "busing dishes at the Renaissance Hotel." She left the rest to my imagination.

After taking a thorough history and giving Julie a physical, I made a plan. The plan consisted of walking calmly out of the exam room and into the office of Rob, my attending, to ask him what to do about Julie. Clearly, as a first-year resident I was in over my head with this patient. Rob sat down with me and went over her general workup. First I should get an MRI of the brain with thin coronal images through the temporal lobes, an EEG, and blood levels. Then I should try high-dose monotherapy with the appropriate anticonvulsant, followed by one or two trials of polytherapy. Finally, if necessary, I should obtain inpatient video/EEG monitoring to see if the patient is a candidate for surgery. Rob thought the monitoring would likely happen sooner rather than later. He offered to help me through the workup. Then he turned, smiled, and said, "Oh, and by the way, please make sure she is not driving, swimming alone, or working in any situation that could harm her, such as around dangerous machines, industrial kitchens, and the like." I looked at him, dumbfounded, then started to speak, but he was gone.

I walked back into the room, excited about "my" plan. It was then that I really learned what I was up against. Julie told me what the plan was before I could get the words out. She didn't miss a beat. She thought it was all a great idea but unfortunately it would have to be put off for a time because she didn't have any money and she had to pay her debts before she would incur any more bills. I looked at her and said, "Julie, how are you going to do that? You've had four jobs in four weeks and you've got a handful of notes in your purse from bill collectors. Why don't you file for medical assistance? We'll get your medicines and all the tests covered. Then we'll have a shot at getting rid of those seizures." Julie looked at me and said, "But then I wouldn't be able to work." This was a determined woman. Her medical chart and the notes from her past physicians read like a Who's Who in neurology. If all those skilled physicians hadn't been able to help Julie very much, the odds that I would succeed in doing so on a first visit were pretty slim. She reluctantly agreed to having her blood levels checked, though we would check them only infrequently to keep costs down. I would try to get her a free EEG in the lab. I threw away her billing sheet, a practice that I later learned was relatively common among residents seeing uninsured patients.

We went to work. The next 7 years passed quickly. Julie came to see me every 3 or 4 months except when she was enrolled in new drug studies. She graciously accepted any chance to try an investigational agent for which she would not have to pay. The protocols, of course, meant that she would have to be up early in the morning and take more bus trips to the hospital, but she didn't seem to mind, although the sleep deprivation sometimes caused her to have seizures in the office. We kept a little stash of medication in the clinic for her and managed to get through the office visits. When I moved to another university-affiliated hospital as an attending, Julie followed me. The bus trip was even longer for her now, but it was the first time she had ever had a resident who had stayed in town. We seemed to bond somehow, and I really looked forward to her visits.

The studies went on and on, but nothing changed. Julie's seizures continued to come, two, three, or even four times a week, although they didn't always become generalized. As the years passed, Julie's memory seemed to become slightly impaired. She sustained an ankle fracture here, a concussion there, and she was starting to tire. The seizures were obviously taking their toll.

Finally, one day Julie came into my office and said, "You know, Dr. Witt, I think you're right. I think it's time I got medical assistance and really had these seizures looked at. If there is a chance that surgery would help me, I'm interested." We made progress quickly over the next several months. Julie continued to have seizures while her medical assistance paperwork went through according to schedule. She had an MRI that showed evidence of right mesial temporal sclerosis, which indicated that she might be a good candidate for epilepsy surgery, after which she might even be seizure-free. Her routine EEG was unclear in terms of localizing her seizures.

After a long discussion with Julie, we made plans to admit her to the Epilepsy Monitoring Unit to record her seizures and see whether they were coming from the scarred region of the right temporal lobe. "Are there any risks?" she asked. "If you have a lot of seizures at one time or a prolonged seizure that needs to be stopped with medication, it could possibly cause some injury," I told her. I went on to tell her that the odds of this happening were small. She said that she trusted me and would stick with whatever plan I thought was reasonable. I assured Julie that the plan was reasonable and that I would continue to be closely involved in her care while she was hospitalized at the university.

At last the day arrived when Julie was admitted. Her medication dosages were tapered gradually, and she began to have occasional seizures. The first couple of seizures were from the scarred right temporal lobe. I was excited because, finally, after watching this young woman suffer for all these years, I had reason to hope that she might be cured of her disorder.

Julie had been in the monitoring unit for about 5 days when I found a note in my office one Monday morning telling me to call the attending or nurse clinician at the unit as soon as I got in. I reached the nurse manager at about 8:30 a.m. She told me that Julie had had a rough weekend and a flurry of approximately 10 seizures, many of which had generalized.

The next few days were really tough. Julie became increasingly confused, and postictal psychosis developed. She became tearful and paranoid and even called the police, believing that the nurse was taking money from her purse. Then Julie's medications were restored.

At the end of her stay on the unit, the monitoring was declared a success. Every seizure had come from the right temporal lobe, so Julie could continue to move through the protocol as a candidate for epilepsy surgery. A few other procedures had to be taken care of, such as Wada testing, neuropsychological testing, and an in-depth discussion of the challenges that might await Julie if she elected to have surgery.

Julie was discharged to her home but continued to be confused. She was placed on low doses of an antipsychotic medication and her mother came from out of state to stay with her. Julie had kept her family at a distance in recent years, ever since she had married a man with whom she did not always get along. The relationship was not good for her and family relations had become strained. Julie's mother, although very caring and concerned, had made a point of not interfering so that Julie could sort things out for herself.

One day the following week, Julie called me at my office. Her voice sounded strange and somewhat distant. "Dr. Witt," she said, "I really hate to disturb you, but I feel really strange, almost as though I'm not here. Actually, the reason I called is because I think I'm dead." The hollowness in her voice sent a chill through me. I understood that postictal psychosis could be severe, but I had never heard a patient utter such words. It frightened me. "Julie," I said, "since you're talking to me, I don't think it's likely that you're dead, but why don't you come see me today with your mom and we'll discuss it." I knew I had to see her in a hurry.

That afternoon, Julie and her mother came into the office, and we talked for a long time. Julie's memory still seemed impaired, even though the monitoring had been completed 2 weeks before. Julie had difficulty recalling recent events, such as her problems in the Epilepsy Monitoring Unit. At least she hadn't any more seizures since her discharge, a new record for her. Julie seemed to understand that since she was able to talk to her mother and me and could feel, see, taste, and hear, she probably wasn't dead. Still, I could tell from her voice that some doubt remained. We discussed the possibility of surgery for her epilepsy and what lay ahead. After about an hour and a half, I felt that it was safe to send her home, and I increased the dosage of her antipsychotic medication. She left in better spirits, promising to call me later in the week.

About 4 days later, while I was planning my schedule for the following day and looking at the picture on my desk of my three little boys, the phone rang. It was a representative from the state epilepsy association. "Dr. Witt," she said, "I have terrible news." The tone of her voice filled me with dread. "What's the matter?" I asked. She replied, "I had been trying to call Julie for 2 days but hadn't gotten any answer, so I brought a policeman with me today to her apartment." "Is she okay?" I asked, my heart beginning to pound. She said, "We broke down the door and found Julie in bed. The paramedics told me she is dead."

I felt as if I had been kicked in the chest. All the wind rushed out of me, and I wasn't able to speak for a time. I then asked, "What happened? Are there signs of violence? Did someone break into the apartment?" She said, "No, she was in bed. She looked as though she was asleep."

As I sit here at my desk a year and half later, thinking back on that day, an empty, hollow feeling comes over me, as it does every time I think of Julie. That young woman trusted me with her life. In my zeal to rid her of her seizures, I tried year after year to convince her to have epilepsy monitoring and perhaps surgery. Everything I had learned from my books and professors told me that this was the right thing to do. Yet Julie had resisted. Did she know something that I didn't know?

Perhaps our role as physicians is not always to do what is *medically* right but to really think about our patients, about what their lives are like, and to strive for a balance between good sense and good medicine. Perhaps having her seizures cured was not something Julie could have endured. All this talk about forced normalization—I'll never know. I look back on that day and I remember crying at my desk when I learned of Julie's death. I will never forget her, and every time I talk to a new patient about epilepsy monitoring or epilepsy surgery, about what we can do to help, she is in the back of my mind. I listen carefully and no longer try to steer patients toward what I think is right. I tell each one of them the first day that my job is to be their advocate, to help them understand all we know about epilepsy now.

I'll never know if Julie's flurry of seizures in the monitoring unit caused her sudden death a few days later, but nothing was found on autopsy to suggest that there was another cause. I'll also never forget the eerie sound of Julie's voice when she called me, predicting her own death.

It is something I'll carry with me for the rest of my life.

59

After a few decades of treating persons with epilepsy, I can remember many inspiring patients and many disappointments. Certain themes, however, run true in my relationships with patients day after day, week after week, and year after year. Even as new tests and medications become available to improve our diagnostic and treatment armamentarium, I am constantly reminded that spending time with patients and their families may be the single most important part of caring for patients with epilepsy.

The introduction of new antiepileptic drugs can be wonderful. It is tremendously exciting when patients either stop having seizures or experience a marked reduction in seizure frequency. When their other antiepileptic drugs are reduced or stopped, other good things can happen. Patients who were usually unable to communicate because of a mental cloud of medication toxicity actually walk into your office and can joyfully tell you how much better they are. These experiences impress you: everything you hear about the importance of quality of life is true.

Other times, though, new drugs bring new problems. Over the years I have learned to temper my enthusiasm for the latest therapeutic procedure, diet, or medication. As a patient's mental faculties brighten and the patient becomes more self-aware, he or she may tell you about disappointments in life and the tremendous burden that epilepsy has imposed. The patient may become angry, depressed, or anxious. To these patients, the new "cure" ironically leads to dissatisfaction.

True, we will rarely be able to satisfy all our patients. Yet the day that we stop caring and being an enthusiastic advocate for any of our patients is the day we rob that patient of hope.

Medicine is an art. The most important and rewarding aspect of practicing this art is the feeling of closeness that you develop with patients and their families. Your patients need not become your best friends, but there must be mutual respect that allows a long-term relationship to develop and flourish. Personality conflicts will no doubt occur with some of your patients and result in noncompliance, being second-guessed, or just feeling as if you are being used. The sooner that you recognize and deal with these issues, the better it is for all concerned. Openly discussing these problems frequently clears the air and strengthens your relationship with the patient, allowing a long-term pact to develop.

Caring for patients with epilepsy requires perseverance, understanding, and patience. For patients with refractory epilepsy, the quick fix is rarely possible. We need to be a counselor for those patients and celebrate in their joys even as we partake in their disappointments. Recently a long-time patient of mine with well-controlled juvenile myoclonic epilepsy became pregnant for the first time. After she discovered the pregnancy she came to me with many questions, all of which I knew we had discussed before. My time, energy, and understanding were again required to allay her fears. Fortunately, the medical aspects of her pregnancy were rather straightforward, and I am happy to report that mother and child are doing well. Her triumph in successfully going through the pregnancy prompted a great celebration for the parents and their extended families. This, my friends, is the joy that caring for people with epilepsy is all about, and we should never forget these times.

I once asked Dr. Kiffin Penry what he looked for in young neurology residents who were interested in the field of epilepsy. He responded that he looked for the fire in their eyes. He knew that the fire burned from a true sense of caring for patients and an energy that never let those physicians settle for second best.

Our charge is to maintain and rekindle that enthusiasm for our patients. Our patients completely place their faith and trust in us. In the memory of Kiffin, we must never let them down.

Providers with Epilepsy

60

(*Psychotherapist*)   By nature, I am not a procrastinator, but as I try to find the words to describe my lifelong experience with epilepsy, I find the task somewhat daunting. And yet, it is really very simple. After all, I have lived with epilepsy all my life.

Living with epilepsy seems ever challenging—sometimes more, sometimes less— but always there. During my adolescence, well-respected and well-intentioned physicians sought 100% control of my seizures. In my twenties, I slowly began to realize that this goal would probably never be realized and I came to accept the chronic nature of my seizure disorder. I did not exactly lose hope; rather, I began to accept the inevitable. Seizures were predictably unpredictable.

For years I would search for the precipitant of each seizure. Then one day I acknowledged that this was a fairly fruitless way to try to bring control over the uncontrollable. What I *could* do was take good care of myself: sleep well, drink none, stay cool, laugh a lot, and always bring coffee to the movies. Other than that, I had to yield to the chemistry of my brain.

I am told that the seizures last a minute or two. Now, most of my seizures occur when I am either drowsy or falling asleep. I know that I have had a seizure during the night if I awake the next morning to find my bed sheets ruffled, things on the floor, and the remnants of my stereotypical reach for the tissue box. If I am awake, the seizure starts with a déjà vu feeling that I refer to as "Oh, no! Here we go again." At that moment I feel invincible, but after recovering from the seizure I remind myself that this was a false sense of invincibility considering there was no stopping the force of my brain's electrical surge. I stare off into space, mumble something incoherently, twitch on one side, lose consciousness and, if the setting is right, drift off to sleep. My seizures are followed by headache and a vague sense of depression, which I believe is both biologic and psychological in origin.

Between seizures I lead quite an average life, but the problem never goes away. It is the last thing I think about before falling asleep and the first thing I think about upon waking up.

My personal life, especially my most intimate life, has been altered immeasurably by virtue of having epilepsy. Relationships are complex to begin with. Add epilepsy and the picture is complicated even more. To that, add the dilemma about having children (risking my child's health) and it is like making chaos out of confusion. So, as I reach my fortieth birthday, it sometimes seems that managing my own life is trouble enough. Despite it all, I enjoy my close friends, love my work, and find passion in everyday living.

I am a practicing psychotherapist. The nature of my work enables me to keep my own personal matters private. The relative anonymity of the therapist makes for sound clinical work. I try not to let my own life interfere with my patients' lives. For this reason, I chose a long time ago to keep my seizure disorder a private affair. This decision also saved me from having to share the humiliating and shame-inducing aspects of my illness with the people I treated.

Having made the decision to keep my epilepsy secret, my work with patients was the one part of my life in which I could pretend that I didn't have a seizure disorder. I felt lucky in that regard. Whereas my colleagues, friends, and family knew the details of my medical history intimately and many of them had seen my seizures, work was my one private domain.

But this past year, for unknown reasons, I had four daytime seizures and my life was turned upside down. Suddenly, driving privileges were taken away from me. I was reminded that driving is a luxury, not a right. Furthermore, my anxiety about having a seizure in front of fragile and vulnerable patients made me realize that I could no longer keep my seizures secret from them. Now, in the interest of high-quality patient care, I had to be open with my patients. My history would have to be shared out of respect for the patients who depended on me.

All my patients came to learn about this part of my life. I had hoped that this would never happen, so that they would not have to be burdened. Yet my patients and I have survived the last year and are probably separately and collaboratively stronger. If I had to do it all over again, would I do it the same way? Possibly yes. Did it deepen our therapeutic relationship and move our work forward in some important way? Probably yes. Do I wish I could have kept it private? *Definitely* yes.

As of this writing, thanks to cutting-edge pharmacology, changes in body chemistry, and whatever other mysteries the brain holds, I seem to be back to baseline. Again I feel like it is my choice to reveal my history and current medical condition. I have acquired some measure of strength from having to cope with the lingering, life-shaping effects of epilepsy, and my own vulnerability and acceptance of my illness have enabled me to help others draw strength from their own personal, and sometimes painful, legacies.

61

(*Physician*)   I spent my twenty-fifth birthday as an intern on the cardiology rotation. I remember two highlights of that day: sharing a birthday cake with the intensive care unit nurses and other residents, and coming home to my husband, who had bought a bottle of Dom Perignon to celebrate.

Everything for me was right on track. I had graduated from college in 3 years in order to enroll in medical school as soon as possible. I was accepted into a prestigious program in internal medicine. I expected to take a fellowship in hematology/oncology after my residency, find a position in academic medicine, and have our first child by the time I turned 34.

One month after my twenty-fifth birthday I woke up in the holding area of my hospital's emergency room. Things were coming off track. Way off track.

The day before, I had taken a walking tour of the city with my husband and a friend. A large chunk of loose paving material was kicked up by a passing car and struck me in the back of my head. At least that's what I was told. My memory of that day stopped abruptly at an earlier point in the day, when we had taken a break from walking to get some ice cream.

I was taken to the emergency room and sent home with pain pills and a directive to take a few days off. A month later I went back to work on a days-only basis until I felt back to normal. After several weeks, I still suffered from headaches, unsteadiness, blurred vision, poor short-term memory, somnolence, and photophobia.

The most difficult thing for me was that, for the first time in my life, my best was not good enough. Yet I felt incapable of trying any harder. My recall of some well-learned facts, such as electrolyte values, was fine. On the other hand, my immediate recall was frighteningly poor. One day I got up from a table in a nursing station to get something and couldn't remember what I wanted. A nurse looked at the chart and asked me if I needed another sheet for my daily note. I did.

The director of the residency program and my fellow interns were very understanding, but one of the chief residents told me in an elevator, "I hope you realize what a burden you are to the other residents." I remember the look on his face as he said that, and the memory of his casual comment still hurts.

On the basis of my ongoing symptoms, the neurologist who had seen me in the emergency room changed his diagnosis from concussion to postconcussive syndrome, advised me to take a leave of absence, and told me that only time would help. When I accepted the leave of absence I knew that I didn't understand what was happening in my head. I was afraid the neurologist didn't understand, either.

My residency program director held an internship slot for me for the following year, but I called him about a month before the internship match day to say he should accept another intern. There was no way I could handle overnight call duty.

One bright spot in the 6 months after the accident was an offhand comment that my husband made late one night. He said, "I hate to admit it, but we've had more time together since the accident than we've had in years." I was shocked that he would dare to find something good in what had happened to me. But then I recalled that I had prayed in the emergency room that I wouldn't die because I didn't want to leave my husband. At that point I wasn't thinking about my career.

Soon I was to became plagued by weird headaches that always began with an overwhelming smell of garlic and proceeded relentlessly to disorientation and lethargy before fading away. My only relief was to lie down and try to sleep. Over the next 5 years I had clusters of these headaches. Meanwhile, I reached a functional plateau that was sustainable but frustratingly lower than my previous level of functioning. I did well in an increasingly demanding series of health communications positions, and I could function at home except before my menstrual periods.

As if that weren't enough, the neurologist always said the same thing at each appointment. "You *should* be improving with time." I felt defensive every time he asked me if I wasn't at least a bit better, and I occasionally felt like crying after appointments because I couldn't shake the feeling that I should have been the doctor, not the patient.

Eventually, I forced the issue of obtaining a second opinion and saw a neurologist who was an expert in head injuries. By the time I had finished my history, he gave me a tentative diagnosis of temporal lobe epilepsy and ordered an EEG (which hadn't been performed before). It showed evidence of a temporal lobe disturbance and I officially became an epileptic.

My husband was very understanding; in fact, he was truly pleased that we had a diagnosis and the hope of therapy. But I felt devastated. It took years before I could let go of the feeling that I was a double failure. I had sustained sufficient brain damage to cause epilepsy and I had been too blind or stupid to analyze my own symptoms when the first neurologist clung to his original diagnosis of postconcussive syndrome.

My family had a surprising (to me) range of reactions. My mother was sure I would be fine if I only had more will power. My father didn't want to talk about my health at all. When I had a seizure during a visit to their home at Christmas, I woke from a postictal nap to hear my mother telling my father that she didn't know how to handle the fact that I had embarrassed them and ruined their afternoon.

For several years my seizures were well controlled on an anticonvulsant, except for an occasional seizure before my menstrual period. Not knowing other women with epilepsy, I thought I had a unique form of premenstrual syndrome.

With fewer seizures, I advanced to other professional positions in health education or communication and my self-esteem improved. My most awkward moments came when I had an appointment with a physician I did not know. He or she would inevitably say something like, "You know a lot about medicine. Are you a nurse or something?" I still feel defensive when explaining my circumstances.

Four years ago, as part of a New Year's resolution to "live better with epilepsy" (whatever I thought that meant), I contacted our state epilepsy organization and joined a support group. I cannot overstate how much I have gained from the unquestioning acceptance of a diverse group of people who all live with epilepsy. I learned that the responses of family members to seizures are often disappointing and negative, even when someone has had epilepsy for a long time. I discovered that medical excellence and medical ignorance are often found in the same institution, and sometimes within the same neurology department. I realized that many people are afraid to say "I don't understand" to their neurologists and that a number of neurologists don't spend the time needed to make sure their patients understand the information or therapeutic options being presented to them. Ironically, I often found myself apologizing for doctors, as if they're cousins but many times removed.

Being in a support group has made me feel blessed that I don't have to live with the fear of grand mal seizures in public places. It is difficult for me to complain about a simple partial seizure or two per day to someone else who is afraid of losing a job because of several grand mal seizures in the workplace within a week. It is impossible, and probably not constructive, to compare the pain of accepting the onset of epilepsy in adulthood with the pain of never having had a normal life.

The most wonderful thing about my experiences in support groups and with an epilepsy organization is that I can personally help the other group members by sharing my rich personal and academic experiences with them. That isn't much different from the goal I set when I decided to become a physician.

I regularly see EEG technicians, nurses, or other health-care workers who ask about my medical and education history. I have met some incredibly understanding and wonderful professionals. In fact, I picked my gynecologist because she was not only competent but knowledgeable and matter-of-fact about epilepsy. She collaborated well with my neurologist, my husband, and me, and thanks to her we have a healthy, beautiful toddler who is a great joy to both of us and, in a way, to my physicians as well.

Yet I have also encountered some amazingly incompetent and prejudiced physicians. After the birth of our son, I had an appointment with a new internist. He called the referring physician to ask whether women with epilepsy "should be allowed" to have children. The internist obviously didn't think so.

Living with epilepsy will always pose a number of challenges. Managing the disorder isn't the most difficult of them. Most difficult is managing my *reaction* to the disorder, especially when seizures are frequent.

I hope that over time I can continue to be active in health education for both lay persons and professionals. I hope that I never get angry and yell at my husband because our lives would have been better if only the accident had never happened. I hope that I am always grateful for the lessons that living with epilepsy has taught me. In fact, I hope that I can always recognize that epilepsy has valuable lessons to teach everyone.

Living with the disorder has brought out many of my best and worst characteristics, made me aware of my strengths and my limitations, and made me appreciate that I am still alive. And, if I am lucky, I will be able to pass on some of this wisdom and understanding to my son when the time comes to explain about Mommy, epilepsy, and the interdependence we all share.

62

❖ ❖ ❖ ❖ ❖

(*Nurse*) One would expect that it would be easy for me, as a nurse specialist in the field of epilepsy, to talk about my personal experi-

ences with epilepsy and how I feel when seizures manifest themselves within me. But it isn't.

Over 10 years ago, when I was a young adult, I received the diagnosis of generalized epilepsy. The neurologic consultant prescribed
anticonvulsant drugs. After 6 months I achieved full control of my
seizures, my future, and my destiny. Or so I thought.

It was important that I gained optimal seizure control because I
was training to be a Registered Sick Children's Nurse. Without complete seizure control I would have been withdrawn from nurse training. Even today, the nursing profession in the United Kingdom still
discriminates against people with epilepsy, in my opinion.

During the first 10 years that I had epilepsy, I never suffered from
the condition because it never minimized my quality of life in any
way. The only problem I experienced resulted from the ignorance of
other nurses, who based their attitudes about epilepsy on old wives'
tales and the old-fashioned stigma surrounding epilepsy. I did not
feel bitter that people had these attitudes; rather, I felt saddened that
they were unenlightened and blind to the truth.

While seizure-free, I could enjoy all that life had to offer me, including employment, a driving license, and a full social life. I felt
that I was in control of my future. Life was good to me. Because I
felt a moral obligation to pay some of it back, I became an advocate
for people with epilepsy. I tried to make the public more aware of the
individuality of the person with epilepsy and of epilepsy itself.

I desired to improve myself academically and worked hard to become qualified in clinical nursing, speech and language therapy, and
science teaching. Professionally I was successful and became a senior university lecturer. This academic position enabled me to further pursue my interest in epilepsy and research. For example, at present I am studying the attitudes and perceptions of young people
with epilepsy in the United States and the United Kingdom.

It would seem, then, that my story is a tale of a person with
epilepsy done good. But I became so engrossed in work, study, ad-
vocacy, and travel that I made one serious mistake: I forgot that I actually had epilepsy.

For too long I had put work first and my health second. Then,
one December, my body decided to remind me that I still had
epilepsy. Initially I ignored the early warning signs, thinking (or

perhaps hoping) that I was imagining it. But I suffered seizures that were frightening and unlike any I had ever experienced before. Fortunately, I was in the United States, staying at a friend's house. My friend assisted me through these terrifying and unusual experiences. To that person I am indebted and will be eternally grateful. And, luckily for me, many people in a wonderful neurology department treated me. To all of them I send my special thanks, should they read this story.

When I first learned that I had epilepsy, I had no direct knowledge of my seizures because I lost consciousness straight away. But before some of my new seizures occurred I felt that something was going to happen, like a sinking feeling in my stomach or bladder. It was as though my body were going to fold in on itself. However, I was unable to verbalize this feeling when it was happening. Even so, my friends could sense that I was switched off from them. They also said that I repeated words or agreed repeatedly if they asked me a question.

Usually in the evening or during the night, I experienced myoclonic jerks of my head, neck, arms, and upper body. I experienced these more regularly if I was very tired or failed to keep a normal schedule. After a tonic–clonic seizure I woke up in the middle of the night aching all over, sometimes bruised, and having urinated. Personally, I hate this type of seizure because I am embarrassed to be incontinent, particularly when I am in somebody else's home. Even though I am a nurse, I am still a person who is personally sensitive and capable of being embarrassed.

At other times, when I was conversing with someone, I either inappropriately continued to answer using the words "yes" or "okay" or I looked ahead as if in a trance and stared. Sometimes my eyelids would flicker and flutter. These trances started instantaneously. If I was stirring something at the stove, I may have put my hand in the hot pan. Sometimes I heard the person instructing me to move my hand and sometimes I could move it. However, when people spoke to me during these trance-like periods, my brain's center for replying seemed to be disconnected from my language area. These seizures were worse when I was in a place with intense sensory stimulation, such as a shopping mall or restaurant. It was as if my brain had just too much to cope with.

Since returning home from a trip abroad, I have been off work for 3 months. Three long and wretched months. I am unable to do my university work and advanced studies because I cannot master the required skills, partly because 3 weeks of intermittent nonconvulsive seizures have left my brain too tired and ineffective to be able to complete the required tasks. My seizure control is improving, but I have learned never to take my personal health for granted again.

The editors of this book initially asked me to write this story 1 year ago. Last year it would have read very differently, perhaps very positively. This year—well, you be the judge.

63

(*EEG technologist*)   I have two types of seizures, both of which, fortunately, are very well controlled.

I have no warning before either type of seizure, and I am unaware during them. I can really remember what happens only after they are over. The first kind, absence seizures, used to occur 30 to 50 times a day when I was a child, and each one lasted 10 to 30 seconds. When I was younger, my eyes would roll back and I would remain motionless and unresponsive. As a child I remember being very embarrassed. I scrambled to make excuses to explain why I couldn't finish my sentences. I was known as the class "space cadet." I told my parents not to tell anyone, not even my grandparents. I couldn't believe there was something wrong with my brain.

Now I only have clusters of absence seizures every 6 months, usually after extreme stress, such as a serious argument or a poor night's sleep. The seizures are only about 2 or 3 seconds long and always occur first thing in the morning. I don't lose my place while talking because they're so short. My husband notices them only if I first tell him that it is one of *those* mornings. He says that my eyes move and look funny for a split second. I can feel my eyes involuntarily move or, all of a sudden, I will find myself thinking about something else with no sense of continuity between the two thoughts. All my life I have likened an absence seizure to a skipping record.

I have also experienced three tonic–clonic grand mal seizures. These occurred as I grew older and as the frequency and severity of the absence seizures decreased. After these seizures I feel completely, totally sad. I don't know why. Perhaps it is part of the postictal state, or perhaps I suddenly realize that I still do have epilepsy even though I live day to day as though I don't have it, apart from taking my medications. This sadness is the worst part, even worse than my tongue hurting so badly and my body feeling so beat up all over after a seizure.

I was given the diagnosis of epilepsy when I was 10 years old. I was completely ashamed and could not believe that someone as average as I could have a disorder of the brain. Up until then I had heard nothing about epilepsy except for crude jokes. At first, I would not take medication. I thought that when kids at school saw me take pills they would laugh and gossip.

Over the years my attitude changed drastically, although I don't know why. I decided not to let seizures get in my way, and in fact I chose to pursue a career as an EEG technologist. I had undergone so many EEGs over the years that it seemed like a great idea. I took a keen interest in my training, joined support groups and epilepsy societies, and attended epilepsy conferences.

Having epilepsy has had a positive effect on the care I give patients. I can understand their angst after the first seizure. I understand how a parent sometimes wants to shelter a child who has epilepsy, but I know how important it is not to do so. I have always had the name of the local epilepsy society and local support group on hand to give to patients. I will correct any myths that I hear about epilepsy. I never tell my patients that I have epilepsy because I just do not feel it is my place. I am there to do a procedure and not to get actively involved in patients' lives. Besides, my experiences do not apply to everyone with epilepsy.

Although epilepsy has never had negative effects on my career, I have been disappointed by the attitudes I have encountered in the workplace. I was told once not to let any of the referring doctors ever find out I had epilepsy because they might not send patients to our

EEG laboratory. If I had a seizure, I might scare the patients away, I was told. Another time an older technologist whom I worked with suggested that I confine my typing to a typewriter because a computer screen might bring on seizures. I do not have photoconvulsive epilepsy and I had been flashing the strobe light during EEGs for patients for years without any problems.

Epilepsy is definitely not the same for all people. That's why I do not like anyone to tell me what I should do about my seizures unless the person is completely familiar with my case. When I tried to join a health club I had to get a doctor's approval. I often wondered what epilepsy meant to those people at the health club. No one asked if I was taking medication, if my seizures were under control, or what kind of seizures I had. Furthermore, no one ever asked what to do if I had a seizure. But to me, none of this mattered. I saw no reason not to be allowed to exercise.

With respect to other aspects of epilepsy and my personal life, I have been very fortunate. My husband has been wonderful. I told him about my seizures as soon as we started dating. He sees my goal of changing societal attitudes about epilepsy as partly his goal as well. He has also made an effort to educate people about epilepsy.

I am also fortunate that my family members and I are close. They have been very good in their attempts to understand epilepsy. They were never overprotective. Ironically, even my parents' dog has seizures. I always loved that dog, and when I found out that she had seizures I loved her more!

Once my husband told me that I was very lucky because my career was so close to my heart. My husband is also in the medical field, but he says that he does not have a similar passion for his work. I realize that not all people with epilepsy want to go into an epilepsy-related field, and that is fine. It might be too much for some people with epilepsy to handle. I appreciate wanting to separate one's personal life from work. But for me, having epilepsy makes everything at work relevant, and it makes me want to go to work.

To this day, I hate seizures being referred to as *fits* and I hate being known as an *epileptic*. I hear many people in the medical field use these two words. I know I am being picky, but the term "fit" is vague and archaic. The terms we use should not perpetuate outdated attitudes. I do not like being referred to as an epileptic, because epilepsy does not consume my life. *Epileptic* is a label and I *refuse* to be labeled and spend my life confined by the parameters of that word.

64

(*Anesthesiologist*)   I was a practicing anesthesiologist. Despite all the admonitions against doctors acting as their own physicians, I diagnosed a seizure disorder in myself. Maybe that was a mistake.

I went to my internist and told him that I was having seizures. I would go into a daze and become forgetful even though I appeared to be talking and walking normally. My internist didn't believe me.

At that time my workload had become heavy, as had the demands on my time at home. Consequently, I was under a great deal of stress. Then, God knows why, I had a grand mal seizure. I was rushed to the intensive care unit because my oxygen saturation was significantly depressed. When I recovered the next day, my internist came and apologized because he had not responded to my pleas for help. His statement was "I guess you were right. You were having seizures." Before that he had said, "It's all in your head."

At home and at work, everyone thought that I was on drugs or intoxicated. No one believed otherwise. And yet I tried hard to explain to anyone who would listen that I was having seizures. I experienced frustration, depression, hatred, and anger toward the world—and toward myself as well.

After a while, I actually started to believe that it *was* all in my head—until I met my neurologist. He was very sympathetic and understanding. Once, he made a joke and said, "Yes it really is in your head, because you are really having seizures." He gave me books to read and for my family to read so that everyone could understand and help me deal with my problems.

The reading helped the situation at home, but things at work deteriorated. Deeper humiliation and frustration set in. My neurologist suggested that I see a counselor to help me understand that I was not the only one with seizures.

My family stood by me, but my seizures worsened and I had to stop working. If that hadn't happened, I probably would have quit my job anyway. My colleagues, who I thought trusted me, tested random samples of my blood for illicit drugs. Given my personality and background, I was devastated.

I admire and adore my neurologist. He made me face these problems and helped me through them. We were unsuccessful in finding medications that worked, except one that carried a substantial risk for serious side effects. It looked as though I was back to square one. I was very forgetful and often in a daze. People had to repeat themselves all the time.

Even though my husband supported me, the truth of the matter was that I had to fight my battles all alone. Yes, it became very lonesome and there were times when I asked God why I was still alive. I don't know how many times I prayed to God to take me away. I was often hurt, frustrated, and depressed to the point of being suicidal. I would begin to believe that I was faking the whole thing, despite the clear evidence of absence status on EEG during one of my prolonged seizures.

What was true? What was reality? I knew that everyone was frustrated with me. At times it seemed as if I had no friends. My parents told me to be more understanding. Others told me that I brought it on myself. Maybe they were right, but what was I supposed to do?

Not too long ago, I went into a long seizure and was found hanging off the roof by one hand. My husband grabbed my other arm and pulled me in through the window, picked me up, and tucked me in bed while my 7-year-old son kept yelling, "Dad, do you want me to call 911?" He was frightened. The next day, when I was alone in my bedroom, the poor little child knocked on my door to see if I was there or had climbed through the window and onto the roof again. I felt so sorry for him and his fear. I hated myself for putting him through that experience, and wondered how I would ever get out of this misery.

Hell broke loose when my husband became angry and said that I used epilepsy as an excuse for everything that went wrong. Sometimes I think that no one realized how hard I was working to be my old self. Believe me, the world has no sympathy when you are sick, especially when you have epilepsy.

There were times when I wanted to run away from everyone and start all over again with a new identity. These feelings made me very angry with myself, and I began to hurt and torture myself emotionally. The mind ruling the body and the body ruling the mind. It's a vicious circle: how could I escape? When I felt so alone, so desperately lonely, I got through it by looking forward to my next appointment with my neurologist.

I certainly want to get back to the practice of medicine. I was in practice for 20 years, worked hard, and enjoyed every minute of it. I cannot believe that I am now on the other side, the receiving end, and that I am having so much difficulty being understood by the medical profession. I guess my patients used to feel the same way. I have a lot more sympathy and understanding for them now.

Now my seizures are under much better control. Despite what I have felt in the past, I now feel that the curtain is rising anew for me and will reveal a new act, a new scene, and a new me. I may never again be a practicing physician but I still intend to be a healer. I won't give up hope. I owe this to myself, my family, and my neurologist. I am sure I will have my ups and downs, but I am not willing to quit or say die. I cannot undermine or underestimate my family's help. We must not let ourselves down.

65

(*Physician*)

MYRIAD THOUGHTS
Each thought
dissolved
into another.
The vacant stare
was filled
with visions
of yesterday.

A film of tear-veiled reality.
Enclosed
in a teardrop
were dreams.
The last fringed curtain
dropped
and myriad thoughts
dispersed forever.

66

(*Nurse*) First of all, I must let it be known that I am a nurse today because of my epilepsy. I had my first grand mal seizure at age 15, which was 12 years ago. I don't recall much of that incident. It wasn't until 4 years later that another one occurred. Again, I didn't remember much about the actual seizure. The following year I had two more grand mal seizures preceded by an aura. I would hear a banging noise in my right ear. It was almost as if two pieces of metal were being hit together. This noise was so distracting that it caused me to turn my head to the right as if to see where the sound was coming from. I would then "wake up," feeling very irritable.

Because of the change in my seizures, my neurologist sent me for an MRI, which showed a tumor in my right temporal lobe. Further testing indicated that all of the seizure activity was originating from the same location as the lesion. The testing required me to be hospitalized for a week so that seizures could be induced. At that time I didn't pay much attention to my nursing care because I wasn't ill.

Two months later I had the tumor removed and spent 10 days in the hospital. The nurses were so caring and supportive that I actually cried the day I was discharged and had to say good-bye.

The summer passed and I returned to college for completion of my senior year, seizure-free, or so I thought. It wasn't until I read *Brainstorms: Epilepsy in Our Words* that I realized I was having déjà vu seizures. With medication changes, these episodes came under control. At that time it was 6 months post-op and I was still receiving outpatient care. I never forgot the wonderful nursing care I received and decided to become a nurse myself.

Two years after the surgery I began taking nursing classes and ironically had two grand mal seizures. Just as before the surgery, I had an aura. Now it was time to try a new medication. I became involved in a drug study, but the drug didn't work well. For the first time I began having simple and complex partial seizures. During those seizures I felt a "rush" in my abdomen that moved up toward my throat. I would then feel nervous and anxious. Sometimes I felt confused and knew I was having a seizure. I remember wanting to stop the seizure and feeling frustrated that I couldn't. Those who know me say I looked the same but sounded as if I were drugged. My fine motor skills were unaffected. On one occasion I was driving when one of these seizures occurred. I didn't remember parking my car where I later located it. I did, however, arrive safely and parked the car perfectly. After withdrawing from the study, I was maintained on one medication at a higher dose. Since then, I have not had a complex partial or grand mal seizure.

I feel I am a great nurse today because I can truly relate to patients' feelings. I am willing to disclose my epilepsy to other people with epilepsy or other potentially disabling conditions. By doing so, I hope these people will realize that all goals are attainable in one way or another. Most important, something good can be made from something bad.

Life between seizures is very normal for me. Although I take an anticonvulsant daily, wear a MedicAlert bracelet, and continue to have simple partial seizures, I am living just like everyone else I know. I am getting married in 3 months to a man who has been through all my medical problems with me. He has seen the majority of my seizures, supported me through the surgery and drug study, and loves me for who I am.

For the most part, having epilepsy has not interfered with my life. I have never been denied employment because of my epilepsy. I am, however, a little apprehensive about disclosing information about my medical condition to potential employers. But that apprehension has begun to fade as a result of my increasing confidence in my ability to perform a job to the fullest. I have had minor seizures at work but have always been able to let someone else know when one was going to occur. Fortunately, I have not had any difficulty keeping jobs, which I feel is largely because of the field in which I work. Medical professionals are more aware and less ignorant of the capabilities of a person who has epilepsy.

All in all, living with epilepsy has not been a problem for me. I guess I have chosen to accept it as a condition I must live with, but I refuse to let it be a handicap.

67

(*Nurse*)   And so it begins again. Will this new treatment be the beginning of the end—the end of my seizures?

One fateful day 15 years ago, my husband and I were planning a game of golf with his business associates. I hadn't felt well for several days. I probably had the flu, I thought, or something I had caught while taking care of the babies in the pediatric acute care unit where I worked as a registered nurse. I remember not feeling like getting out of bed the morning of the game, but I did, got dressed, and went outside to wait while my husband, Dan, loaded the clubs into the car. I felt worse as we headed out. About 10 minutes later Dan was talking to me and I could hear him but I couldn't move or answer him. I felt as though I had tipped way over to the side, but when I opened my eyes, I was sitting up straight. It passed and we continued. But then it happened again and again over the next 20 minutes or so. We decided that the golf game would have to wait and headed for the hospital. This experience was very frightening to both of us.

At the hospital, I was supposed to sign papers so I could be evaluated in the emergency room. I had a lot of trouble writing. My signature looked like the scribbling of a child. The doctor did the usual neurologic exam and ordered blood to be drawn, as well as skull x-rays and a computed tomography scan. He told me he would call my internist. Through all of this, the strange "episodes" continued.

There were several other people there. One was trying to pass a kidney stone. Another was in premature labor. One had been in a car accident, and yet another had chest pain. To pass the time, my husband and I (in between spells) tried to guess who would be admitted and who would be sent home. I was hoping that I would get a prescription to stop these episodes and be sent home so I could go to bed. One by one the other patients were discharged and I was the only one left. I was told that I was going to be admitted so they could do a few more tests. Okay.

The next morning, the doctor told me I had complex partial seizures and started me on an anticonvulsant. A neurologist came in later that day and switched me to a different medication. After a week in the hospital, I was discharged.

I had to stay out of work for about a month. I was doing well, so I was given the go-ahead by my neurologist to return to work and resume driving as long as I didn't have any more seizures. When I got back to work, I minimized the whole situation to my fellow nurses.

Then, one evening, I was driving home from visiting a friend when I found myself on a one-way road in a forest, not knowing how I got there. I had another seizure the next day and was told to stop working (and driving). After all, at work I took care of babies on ventilators, babies with tracheotomies, and babies with central lines: very sick babies. It would be more than a little dangerous if I became unresponsive at work. My supervisor said that she would keep my job for 3 months and wished me a speedy recovery. That was the last time I worked in over 4 years. I still grieve over the loss of my job.

Over the past few years I have had many seizures in many places. My husband describes my seizures as being as if someone pointed the remote control of a video cassette recorder at me and put me on pause. I stop whatever I am doing, wherever I am doing it. Someone else described me as being like a mannequin. The seizures last from less than a minute to a couple of minutes, but I can't judge how long they last. Sometimes I estimate a seizure's length by what has gone on around me or what has transpired on television. During a seizure my eyes are closed and I feel as though I am leaning forward or sideways, though I am actually straight. Sometimes I know I am going to have a seizure because I have a funny feeling in my stomach.

Other times I have no warning. Afterwards, I have trouble walking, talking, or doing anything for a little while.

It could be said (tongue in cheek) that seizures are not good for your health. One day I wanted to light a fire in the fireplace. I got everything ready and sat on the raised hearth. I lit the match and touched it to some paper. Then I had a seizure. I couldn't move, and I couldn't see what was happening. I could feel the heat and hear the crackling of the burning paper and kindling, but I could not pull my hand back. A few minutes went by before I was able to move. Luckily I was not burned, but I was upset.

Another time, I was at the sink. I turned the hot water on and put my hands under the faucet, waiting for the water to warm up. Again, I had a seizure and couldn't pull my hands back. This time I did burn my hands because the water quickly became hot.

Most people have been very understanding and helpful to me, but not everyone. One time I had quite a few women at my house for a meeting. While I was in the kitchen I suddenly felt that I was going to have a seizure, so I leaned against a railing to be safe. Two of the women saw me and made a big commotion. They said they had to pull me away from the railing because I might fall over. They were whispering loudly, as if I couldn't hear them. They pulled a chair over and forcibly pushed me down into it. Everyone came running, and I was very embarrassed.

My neurologist has always been kind to me, although at times I think he had doubts about whether I did have seizures. Yet he kept pushing for more answers and effective treatments. Once he told me about a new medication, not yet approved in the United States, that had helped many people and just might help me. I was very optimistic and made an appointment to return in several months when the drug was expected to be available.

As I waited for that appointment, I got more and more excited. So did my family, my friends, and the people at church, who were very concerned about me and the episodes. At that time I did not call them seizures, not even to myself. After all, it might turn out they were something else. I was sort of in denial. Sort of.

In anticipation of this wonder drug, I started to make plans. I hadn't been able to drive or work in 3 years. I planned it all out. I'll start the new drug, spend a few months getting the dose regulated, and by Thanksgiving I will be able to drive! I will spend a whole week driving places I haven't been able to visit. I will take my friends out—the ones who have been giving me rides. I will spread the good news that I don't have to worry about the episodes anymore. Freedom again. Freedom from seizures. Freedom from fear. Freedom from danger. Freedom from embarrassment.

When the day of the appointment arrived I got dressed up, as if I were going to a very special meeting. Nylons, heels, a good dress. The whole bit. I got there early. When my neurologist took me into his office, his first words were, "I'm sorry. The drug is not available yet. Maybe it will be this fall." He said that he would call me when it was available. I think he was almost as disappointed as I was.

I went home. Up to this time, I had gone through many hard times and had kept up a positive attitude. Everyone said so. I had shed a few tears, but only a few. I knew this nightmare would end and life would return to normal. I had made the best of things. I had listened to the rain. I had watched the snow fall. While I was waiting to be picked up to go somewhere, I listened to the birds. I had even read some books. When I was working and leading a normal life, I was far too busy to do these things.

But now my dream was taken away. When I got home, I had a big pity party for myself. No one was there to share it or shed some tears with me. I cried a lot.

Pretty soon, a friend called to ask me how the appointment went. I told her, "Rotten!" She said, "You just have to be patient." Sure. She invited me to go along on an outing. I said, "No, you go. I'll just sit here in my misery. I won't be good company, anyway." Oh, woe was me. Maybe I was overreacting a little. Maybe a lot. My friend insisted I go along. She said it would be good for me. She was going out with another friend, Mary, to buy a dog. Bear with me, now. This is all relevant.

We went to each of the dog pounds in the area. No luck. I sat in the back of the car and didn't contribute much to the conversation. I cried a few more tears, which they ignored.

Off to a pet store. As soon as we got inside, I saw a beautiful white puppy. I fell in love. I held her, and all the tears that had been stored up for 2 years were released. I said I would take her. Juneau (the dog) was going to make me happy.

And she does. When I can't go somewhere because I don't have a ride, Juneau is there to keep me company. When I don't feel well, she is by my feet. When I have a seizure, she puts her head on my knee, sometimes even before the seizure starts.

The "wonder drug" did finally become available, and at first it was a great help to me. My seizures decreased steadily. I cautiously started to think that my timetable for recovery had been only delayed. I used the word *cautiously* because I knew I couldn't get my hopes up too high again. It was too far down to the pits of despair. And besides, one dog was enough.

Some months later my seizures had increased again and I was getting terrible headaches. So much for the wonder drug.

Many other medications came and went. Nothing worked. I was sent to a university hospital for more testing. A psychologist came in, said "Hi," and gave me a paper with 200 questions. Every question had to be answered with a yes or no, even if I didn't know the answer. If the question could be answered correctly with both responses, I had to pick one. Then the psychologist took the paper and counted up the yes's and no's and concluded that I was a person who might under some circumstances have seizures that weren't real. I was devastated. God bless my neurologist for ignoring this conclusion.

I was sent to another psychologist, who spent a day testing me. Her report said that I did not have the emotional makeup or whatever to make up anything about seizures. I was not malingering. In her opinion, the seizures were true seizures. I felt very validated by this report. I didn't want or need the extra pain of not being believed.

Then I was admitted to a different teaching hospital. I found that EEG telemetry with sphenoidal electrodes was as pleasant as walking barefoot in the Sahara desert. I was wired and wrapped up. Surveillance started. Because of marvelous technology, my EEG readouts could be read instantly by a computer down the hall. I thought clean thoughts.

The little monitor high up on the wall allowed my every movement to be observed at the nursing station. The electrode wires were connected to the wall by a leash that was long enough to reach the bathroom. It was comforting to know that if I had a major seizure, help was very close by. My seizure medications, all of them, were gradually reduced over a week. As they were reduced, I had more seizures, but there was no correlation yet with the EEG findings.

About the tenth day, one of the epilepsy doctors came in to see me just as I was having a seizure. He checked the EEG and confirmed that there was a definite correlation between the two. Again, I felt validated. The key to seeing the EEG correlate to my seizure was for me to be completely off seizure medications. That hadn't been done at the other center. Medicines were restarted, and I made plans to go home.

Over the next couple of months, I was given additional combinations of seizure medicines, but I did not get better. Now, I am back to the part about waiting for "it." The beginning of the end of my seizures, I hope.

Because all seizure medications had failed, I became a candidate for a nerve stimulator that is implanted in the upper part of the chest. My husband and I decided to proceed and the surgery was performed. I have a little magnet that I carry with me most of the time. The magnet can be used to activate or shut off the device. I carry it in my pocket or in a cloth pocket around my wrist. It is funny to be eating at a restaurant and find that my knives and forks are sticking to my wrist. Once when I was in a rush, I dropped the magnet in my purse and wiped out all my credit cards. My husband was thrilled, of course.

At this time, I am waiting for the results from the device to become evident. It may take a few months to know if it will be successful. It appears that the device is helping because I am having only a few seizures each month. However, I have been through good periods before, and I want to make sure that the seizures won't return down the road. I am optimistic. I very much want this to work.

Is this the beginning of the end—the end of my seizures?

68

(*Nurse anesthetist*)　　I am a Certified Registered Nurse Anesthetist and married to an anesthesiologist. When we moved East to start a family, I stopped working to be home with my children. Then, when I was 42, epilepsy developed. That was 4 years ago. The etiology of my seizures is unknown. I did have minor head injuries at the ages of 10 and 38, but I did not lose consciousness either time.

I have both generalized and partial seizures. Before a generalized seizure I have no premonition or warning. During the postictal period I always feel tired, confused, and very depressed. These seizures scare me because they can happen anytime and anywhere. For example, I had my first generalized seizure while I was talking on the telephone.

The partial seizures vary. Sometimes I will suddenly come to and realize that a period of time has elapsed. Frequently, after I black out I have tremors in my right hand and drooping of my right eyelid. At other times, after I black out I have involuntary movements on one entire side of my body (according to witnesses).

I also get different types of auras, which are like feelings of foreboding. I call one type a "whoosh." I feel that the bottom is dropping out of my world or that the circulation (especially to my head and legs) has temporarily stopped. It feels as if I will fall if I don't sit down quickly. After this type of aura I have to sit down wherever I am—on the kitchen floor, in the middle of the sidewalk, or wherever there is solid ground. I call another type of aura that I get "the stupids." I have trouble figuring out the simplest things. I can't sequence, retrieve words, construct sentences, or make decisions.

I have other symptoms that do not seem to fit into any category. These include shaking of my head and limbs without loss of consciousness, panic attacks, and mood swings that occur with amazing swiftness. I can go from a good mood to being very depressed in what seems like a heartbeat.

Over the past 4 years I have lost a great deal in my life. I have lost fine motor skills in my hands and fingers. I have lost my self-confidence. I feel that I have even lost the respect of my children. From one minute to the next, they don't know if they'll be talking to the "stupid" mom, the "spacey" mom, the "inconsistent" mom, or the "normal" mom. My younger son brushes me off, and my older son teases me.

But most of all I have lost my independence. This has been the most significant loss to me. For almost 2 years after my seizures began, I didn't go anywhere alone. I didn't even take my dog for a walk. I was afraid of having a seizure in public, afraid of falling down, afraid of getting confused or lost, afraid of embarrassing myself, afraid of becoming incontinent, and afraid that no one would help me.

I haven't driven a car in 4 years, and to me that has been a major inconvenience. As a society, we rely heavily on driving. When you suddenly can no longer drive, a lot of pressure is placed on others to drive you places. In my case, my husband picks up the slack. I truly miss just being able to get in my car and go.

Who can relate personal experiences with epilepsy without including something about seizure medications? As someone who has been involved in health care, I understand the hows and whys of medications. But this knowledge doesn't make it any easier for me to take them.

Up until recently I had trouble with each of the seizure drugs I was prescribed and, besides, none of them stopped my seizures. Fortunately, I have the best seizure control yet on my current regimen. My friends and family say that I have "awakened" on this combination of seizure drugs after so many years of side effects. I can do things again—simple things, for sure, but at least I am getting out and getting on with my life.

It would have been terribly difficult, if not impossible, to work as a nurse anesthetist these past 4 years. Transportation would have been my first obstacle. Scheduled daytime work would have been manageable but working at night would have been difficult. The loss of fine motor skills I suffered would have compromised my ability to start intravenous lines and other lines.

I have always felt that giving anesthesia is an art. An anesthetist acquires the necessary knowledge and skills through education and practice, but the actual administration of anesthesia is often based on a spur-of-the-moment decision. Considering that I have had trouble deciding if I should put on my right or left shoe first, how could I decide which medications to give to a patient in a high-pressure situation? As an anesthetist, you literally control a patient's life. What would happen to the patient and the surgical team if I became confused or had a seizure while administering an anesthetic? Given this risk, I definitely think that I would have resigned if I had been employed when my seizures started. In good conscience, it would have been my only option. The one saving grace is that my husband shares his daily experiences with me. This at least keeps me thinking about anesthesia.

Despite everything I have been through, I have much to be grateful for. I am grateful that I am in a position where I do not have to work and can concentrate on getting my health back, grateful for the love and support of my husband, and grateful for the help of my neurologist.

69

(Nurse)   I have taken care of people with seizure disorders for the past 5 years. I find it challenging to take a seizure history from a new patient, and I know first-hand that this same process can be quite disconcerting. I went through the same turmoil when my own seizure disorder was first diagnosed.

My first overt seizure was 16 years ago, but I believe there may have been other seizures even before that. My mother reminded me of a "fainting spell" I had had on Easter Sunday 2 years earlier. That morning I abruptly awoke and felt exhausted. While showering, I started to feel lightheaded, the room began to spin, and then I blacked out. My mother was in the kitchen. She heard a loud thump and rushed upstairs to the bathroom to find me slumped over and face down in the tub. When I awoke, my head and right hip were bruised and sore. I went to the emergency room to be evaluated and was then released without further treatment.

For the next 2 years I had intermittent blackouts. They were especially embarrassing when they happened while I was on the telephone with friends. Then came the first clear seizure. We were going to Bermuda for a vacation. I was so excited I could not sleep. When we finally reached the hotel I had to nap before dinner. Later, I abruptly awoke and jumped out of bed to shower. I made it as far as the foot of the bed before I blacked out. My poor grandfather saw me fall and strike my head on the bed frame. Then he saw me have a tonic–clonic seizure. The next thing I remember was a pounding headache. My tongue was lacerated. I was irritable and overwhelmed. All I could think about was sleeping. My parents helped me back into bed and I slept. By the next morning I felt much better and was able to enjoy the rest of the vacation without problems.

My parents thought I should be evaluated when we returned home. The first doctor I saw was an old friend of my father's. Initially, I had an EEG and CT scan and was placed on a seizure medication. The sedation was hard to tolerate, even though my level was not yet "therapeutic." My dose was increased and I became extremely sedated. The doctor started to question my compliance. I was subjected to repeated EEGs every 6 months, frequent blood draws, and office visits. I found it difficult to tolerate this evaluation process because I was not having seizures. I grew disheartened with my caregiver and sought another practitioner. My father suggested the names of a few specialists, but they performed similar evaluations and seemed to have the same approach.

I kept searching for answers. What was my prognosis? But I got nowhere. Altogether, I saw five neurologists before growing so frustrated that I decided to see an epileptologist at a comprehensive epilepsy center. He knew how to take an approach that met my needs. I had been looking for this for 6 years! After I received the answers to the questions I had pondered for so long, I was immediately put at ease. For the first time, I felt that I was a part of a team and that I was empowered to make things better for myself.

I have been seizure-free since then, continue to see an epileptologist, and am still taking seizure medication. My experiences strike a chord in me whenever I care for people at our comprehensive epilepsy center. As a result, I strive for excellence in the care I render to people who, like me, have epilepsy.

70

(*Nurse*)   I suffered subdural and epidural hematomas 6 years ago after being struck in the head by a softball during a coed game. I underwent a craniotomy to evacuate the hematomas, and a seizure disorder developed as the result of my injury. For a 2-year period after my injury, I struggled as my physicians attempted to get my seizures under control. Currently, my seizures are controlled with a medication that I take four times daily. My doctor has told me that it is unlikely that I will ever be able to wean myself from this medication.

During the 2 years that my seizures were uncontrolled, I suffered a number of partial seizures and one generalized tonic–clonic seizure. Most of my seizures were preceded by an aura, consisting of a sense of dread and the feeling that adhesive tape or a strand of hair was on the corner of my mouth or on the top of the fingers of my right hand. Unfortunately, not all my seizures were preceded by auras; on those occasions I had no warning of the oncoming disaster. When auras did occur, though, they could be helpful. Once I was swimming in the city pool with my 3-year-old child and felt the aura. I was able to get both of us out of the water and into the locker room, where I seized (safely).

Okay, enough already! Just remembering those days makes me feel uneasy. Now, when I am wrapping a present or blow-drying my hair and adhesive tape or hair happens to attach itself to my fingers, I freak but then smile and say, "No, it's not a seizure, it's actually tape (or hair)."

My epilepsy has affected every aspect of my life. Back when my seizures were uncontrolled, my husband and I attended two hockey games a week apart. At both games I seized and had to go to the first aid station to recuperate. After the second seizure, the security guard outside the door looked up at us, smiled, and quipped, "Why don't the two of you stay home next time and watch the game on TV?" Although his statement was said with good intentions, my husband and I seriously considered his suggestion. Another time I called some friends to ask them out to a movie. Imagine the embarrassment I felt when I was forced to say, "Okay, when will you pick me up?" The inability to drive in and of itself has caused all sorts of practical problems. I have lost my independence, privacy, and general freedom. Try Christmas shopping with an escort.

Now then, let me turn to my epilepsy and my professional career. I'm a circulating nurse in an operating room. When I come upon a patient who has a history of epilepsy or who takes an anticonvulsant, I always ask, "When was your last seizure?" If they answer "Two years ago" or "Ten years ago," the two of us high-five and I yell, "Four for me!" Then the two of us carry on like we're old pals. I hope they feel they can relax and trust me because we have something in common, but I also wonder if they ever question whether I can do the job.

I prefer not to take calls or work after scheduled hours because I have been told that lack of sleep and/or an irregular daily routine could lead to a seizure. I fear that if I'm working and have a seizure, my co-workers might have to stop the surgery and attend to me. I make up the on-call requirements of my job by working two Saturdays out of every six. Obviously this schedule cuts down on the time I can spend with my family on weekends, when they are always home.

I am also fearful about how others will view my epilepsy, including prospective employers. As a result, I have settled into my job at a small, local community hospital, where I have worked for 9 years, 6 of which have been since my accident. It seems likely that I will remain there for the rest of my career.

Although my life has been dramatically changed, I am thankful to be alive, thankful that I am employable, and thankful that I have been able to continue my life in a relatively normal fashion.

71

(*Nurse*)   I never wanted to work in the field of epilepsy. Why should I? I had to live with it every day, and to live and breathe seizures 24 hours a day is neither easy nor fun, to say the least. However, my friend and mentor in graduate school convinced me that I had a special understanding of seizures that others could not possibly have. She persuaded me that I could truly make a difference in the lives of other people with epilepsy. And so began my journey to both live and work with epilepsy.

After a few years in this field, I found myself in the same situation that most of my patients face. I was a scared patient undergoing lots of tests and medication changes and not getting many answers.

Being a nurse made it more difficult for me, contrary to what I expected. Although I had ready access to experts and often received preferential treatment in the scheduling of tests, people assumed that I understood everything and that I could handle it myself. And I thought so, too. Yet the unpredictability and unknowns of my condition became too much for me. My colleagues believed that I had no problems and didn't really need help. The facade that I had worked so hard at putting on was working too well, and now that facade created a barrier to my receiving the help that I really needed.

No, I couldn't do it all by myself. But how could I ask for help to cope and live with seizures when none was offered? Asking for help can be difficult if you also work in the field. Either people assumed I knew more than I did, they didn't listen to what I really said and felt, or they doubted what I said. Being doubted and not believed was one of the worst experiences I have ever had. The next worst one was being believed too much by doctors who perceived me as an all-knowing expert on epilepsy!

Another problem for me during this difficult period was that I was being compared with other patients on our epilepsy unit. Our unit cares for people with seizures that are very difficult to diagnose and treat; in addition, they often have behavioral, psychiatric, or social problems. For those of us who work in the unit every day, it became easy to imagine that everyone with epilepsy worthy of professional attention has such significant problems. We also came to believe that anyone with epilepsy not serious enough to merit an inpatient evaluation didn't deserve any consideration beyond the basic cursory office visit. I was my own worst enemy in this regard. I felt I had no right to complain or feel sad. As a result, I minimized and ignored my own life with seizures.

Computed tomography and MRI scans, endocrine workups, and EEG and neuropsychological testing may be considered simple evaluations to go through, but I still worried about the results. Did I pass? What did the results mean for me? What was wrong? Would I still be able to work? I experienced all the fears and fantasies that many of my patients had expressed to me. I thought how bizarre and crazy this all was. Then I looked around and realized that this was life as usual for so many of my patients. I had been lucky to have been spared these difficulties up to now.

Dealing with people's attitudes about seizures has also been hard for me. Humor is commonly used on our unit as a coping mechanism. Humor can help us face feelings or situations that are out of our control or that feel uncomfortable. Many of my patients and I use humor in this way and feel good that we can do so. But humor can also hurt and be destructive. Jokes about seizures aren't funny if you live with seizures yourself.

I have found that I need to separate my personal experiences with seizures from those of my patients. Empathy and understanding are helpful, but overidentification can be harmful to the treater and the patient. For years I struggled with the stress of finding the right balance. Every morning I prepare myself to see patients by separating my personal issues from my job. Then every night I put away the work issues and put myself back together so that I can cope with the way my epilepsy affects my family and me. This is easy when my seizures are under control. But at other times it can be very difficult and exhausting! Counseling and support from friends who are not involved with epilepsy has helped give me a chance to talk and think in safe places.

It is much easier for me now. I have been lucky—my seizures have been well controlled, although surprises do happen. I know what I feel comfortable about and where my difficulties lie. I can recognize when my personal life is getting in the way of my work and when I need to step back and get some help. And I have learned that I need more time outside of work that has nothing to do with seizures!

Over the years I have learned a lot from my colleagues and from the people I have cared for, and I would like to extend a special "thank you" to everyone I have been privileged to know and to work with. I learned that it is okay to feel sad and to complain. And it is even okay to ask "Why me?" at times. I learned to grieve for how my seizures affected my life. Only then could I live with my epilepsy and feel okay about it. I still may not like it, but I can live with it.

I hope that everyone who works with people with seizures realizes the importance of helping their patients work through their feelings.

Please, take the time to listen to what your patients say and how they feel, and look at your own feelings as well.

There are many people out there counting on you for help.

72

(*Mental health counselor*)   My early experiences with epilepsy definitely shaped me as a person and influenced my decision to become a licensed mental health counselor and to attain a master's degree in counseling psychology. It is no coincidence that I am in a profession in which listening, mirroring, and responding to the angst and fears of others is vital.

I grew up with complex partial seizures. The etiology was unknown. I would wander from point A to point B without knowledge of how I got there. The frequency of my seizures became unmanageable when I was in college, even though I faithfully followed my medication regimen. My self-doubt and the stress of managing a chronic illness required a lot of my energy and focus. I wondered if I would ever be married and have children, let alone complete a graduate degree. The daily management of my epilepsy was my top priority and the rest of my life revolved around it.

Only after I crossed a major traffic intersection on foot during a seizure, unscathed but later emotionally shaken, was I told that brain surgery could help me. I faced this prospect with each of the emotions that Elizabeth Kubler-Ross describes in her book *On Death and Dying*. At first I was angry. I bargained. I doctor-shopped. And then I finally came to accept that surgery was the only option left if I was to pursue my dream of being a therapist. I reasoned that I could make a gain only with surgery, having already lost part of myself to the seizures. After working through these many emotions, I successfully endured 8 hours on the operating table, semiconscious. Now, looking back, I do not know if I would ever have the courage to go through it all again.

Epilepsy made successfully completing undergraduate and graduate schools a challenge. All along I wanted to reach for the stars. And I did. I came up shining, because I was the only person in my family to attain a master's degree. I am proud of this accomplishment given the obstacles I faced.

Having epilepsy also gave me unique opportunities for self-awareness and growth. My struggles made me an empathetic therapist, able to appreciate the worry, pain, and shame that patients often bring into the therapy room. I have learned first-hand that a kind, listening, responsive person can empower another to take control and accomplish the steps necessary to lead a full and challenging life. I apply this realization from my own journey to my approach with my clients. I also have learned from my epilepsy to treat the whole person and to consider the possibility that a patient's symptoms may have an organic basis. I am keenly aware of the role that head injury and genetic constitution may play in a person's manifestation of mental illness or anxiety. My goal in working with patients is to help them realize what they have control over and to tackle these obstacles one at a time.

I have not found my epilepsy to be a deterrent to finding or maintaining work. But there are times when I am hesitant to disclose my seizure disorder to co-workers for fear that they will judge me as less able to carry my load. In some ways, I feel I must first *prove myself* before making any such disclosure. People hold preconceived ideas about epilepsy. I remember a psychologist colleague who, after learning I had epilepsy *and* children, asked, "Do your kids have epilepsy, too?" This type of question is born out of ignorance, but the fact it was even asked unnerved me. I know that in some arenas I am judged as "the woman with epilepsy." But I hope that I will also be known as a woman who cares deeply about her patients and treats them with respect and dignity.

Now, having been seizure-free on medication for 21 years and a parent of two children, my eyes are cast on pursuing my dreams of doing research and improving the lives of those with epilepsy. I find that I am well equipped to manage the tugs and pulls of my professional and personal life, perhaps because I was trained for many years in juggling life with an active seizure disorder.

I am proud to have survived the battle with epilepsy. I know that I have epilepsy, but I also know that epilepsy does not have me.

73

(*Nurse*)   It's hard to know where to begin. I am now 34 years old and have had epilepsy for half my life. My first seizure occurred when I was skiing. All I could remember was falling down very hard and rolling, and then, barely, waking up in the hospital.

My life changed forever after that event that I could hardly remember, although at the time (maybe because of my age) I certainly didn't act like anything had happened. I continued to smoke pot, experiment with other drugs, and drink alcohol.

I underwent the usual barrage of tests. My doctor concluded that I had a seizure disorder. I couldn't even call it epilepsy back then. I was put on seizure medication but took it only when the mood struck me. I was what we in the medical field call a noncompliant patient. I ignored my physician's instructions not to drive a car, and my parents backed me up. Maybe we were all in denial.

Soon my seizures came more frequently. I would become extremely light-headed and try to get help from someone before I collapsed and lost consciousness. I would emerge from the seizure extremely disoriented and would feel normal only after awakening from a deep, postictal sleep. Except that after waking up there would be the inevitable flood of tears. Having a seizure was like losing a piece of your life. What was going on with my body?

Yet I still continued my counterproductive lifestyle. One time I was at a party with my boyfriend. We were snorting cocaine and drinking alcohol. I was told later that I was listening to someone talk who had a particularly annoying voice and I cursed at her, telling her to shut up. I don't even remember the ride home. As I write this story, I am struck by how I now remember experiences such as this one. For a long time I told people that I would lose consciousness only for a few seconds after a seizure. Maybe that was true some-times, but there were quite a few other times, as in this incident with my boyfriend, when I lost my memory for hours!

My neurologist told me that if I went 5 years without seizures and my EEGs were normal, we would discuss taking me off my medica-tion. I became more compliant with my medicine and adjusted my lifestyle for the better. The 5 years came and went. During that time I went to and graduated from nursing school.

I had begun my new career as a nurse when I approached my neu-rologist about coming off the medication. He was hesitant, saying that because I was healthy and doing well he did not think it was a good idea. I decided to seek a second opinion and saw a doctor at the same institution where I worked. After taking my history and re-viewing my records, he was agreeable and weaned me off the medi-cation. Three months later I had a seizure. I started a different med-ication and have been on it ever since.

I did pretty well for several years. Then I came under quite a bit of stress at work and had another event and became extremely disori-ented. I was referred to a new neurologist, who immediately came up to the cardiology clinic where I worked. My other doctors were all very nice, but none showed the kindness and compassion that this neurologist did. He very firmly explained the state law about driv-ing: 6 months without a seizure before I was considered well con-trolled. But, as usual, I went on driving (denial is a powerful thing).

I was in counseling therapy at the time. When I told my therapist about my physician's advice about driving, she told me I'd better call someone to pick me up. I began to cry. I told her I could drive home. I promised her I would drive my car home and would not drive for 6 months. But she was firm. If I drove my car home she would no longer treat me, she said. It was a very painful moment but one I will always thank her for.

I know that there are many people out there who are driving and risking their lives and the lives of others because they, too, deny their epilepsy. I am not saying it's easy. As a matter of fact, it stinks! I am now less than 1 month away from driving again. I've been through this more than once. It is difficult to become dependent on others, es-pecially when you ask someone for a ride and the person turns you down or slowly says, "W-e-l-l, I kind of had plans." Then you feel like a real idiot and hurriedly assure the person, "It's okay, I'll find a way home." Then of course I go into my office and cry. We are all allowed to feel sorry for ourselves once in a while, aren't we?

My husband, Stan, is very supportive. He is adamant that I abide by the state law. He drives me to work almost every day. My last seizure occurred 5 months ago, while we were swimming in the ocean. I lost consciousness and keeled over in the water. Stan saved my life! That night, after we got back from the hospital, Stan just sobbed. He had worked so hard taking care of me all day and was finally able to deal with his own feelings of panic and the prospect of nearly losing his wife.

Stan and I talk about having a baby soon, but he told me that he is concerned about me driving while I'm pregnant. That started the tears flowing again. My 6 months are almost up. I've done my time! *I want to drive again.* But the tears are also tears of happiness. I'm very lucky to have a man who cares about me so much. I thank God for him all the time.

I am the nurse manager of a busy cardiac catheterization lab. I have a very full and active life with lots of love and support from family and friends. It's still not easy having epilepsy. It's been a long road going through the grieving process. But maybe I've truly reached the stage of grief called acceptance. Or maybe I'm as close to acceptance as I will ever get. I still have pity parties sometimes.

Writing about my epilepsy has been very therapeutic for me and has also unearthed some memories that I didn't even know existed. As both a health-care professional and a patient, I can really see the importance of a good support system, not only from family and friends but from the medical community as well.

74

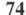

(*Pediatrician*)   Toward the end of World War II, I was blown out of a jeep and ended up on my helmeted head. There were no immediate sequelae.

About 12 years later (and 3 years after getting married) I had my first seizure. According to my wife, it was a grand mal seizure. It was nighttime, and we had just seen *On the Waterfront*. The second seizure, which was similar, happened about a year later. My wife had me seen by a host of physicians and neurologists. I was having occasional auras, along with abdominal cramps, and made peculiar noises. These symptoms gradually decreased, and I eventually returned to normal. Later, I had episodes while driving my car and parked at the side of the highway for no reason. This type of episode happened a few times (twice a month) when my children were in the car with me. The neurologist quickly diagnosed my condition as complex partial seizures. I was 35 years of age, and the seizures were localized to the left temporal lobe by EEG. Recently, when I had a stroke at age 70 (diagnosed as a right pontine infarct), CT and MRI scans revealed an old hematoma in the left temporal lobe, presumably from my war injury.

My first treatment was phenobarbital. Visits to several neurologists and two psychiatrists failed to decrease the severity and frequency of my seizures. Thanks to my wife's observations, I began to realize that the majority of my seizures occurred at night and were recorded by me as abdominal cramps. Initially, I was severely bothered by the diagnosis and by my inability to drive. I felt that I was losing control of my life and my leadership in family matters. I felt ashamed, embarrassed, and confused by the seizures, which left me not knowing what had happened or where I was. The loss of the leadership role turned out not to be as upsetting as I had anticipated, but the inability to drive my own car seemed to me a huge blow.

I advanced through the rank of academic positions to become a full professor in our department and performed research projects that led to my becoming an associate research professor in another clinical department. I was able to proceed with lectures, rounds, and others tasks, and continued to drive until relatively recently. Then, about 40 years after my initial seizure, a rare daytime seizure affected me sufficiently so that my department chairman felt I should no longer be seeing patients, and I therefore gradually withdrew from the clinic and private practice.

I owe the description of my seizures to my wife, who is a witness to them. They almost always occur at night. I cannot recall them except as abdominal cramps. Apparently I make small, generalized movements and, rarely, have a grand mal seizure with loss of urine and/or biting of the tongue or cheek. Regardless of the mildness, severity, or length of the seizure, it is followed, almost always, by severe drowsiness that can last 1 to 2 hours, half a day, or even a full day. Frequency and urgency of urination almost always follow the seizure.

My seizures used to occur about once a week, but my present drug regimen has reduced these nighttime seizures to only once every 2 to 3 weeks. Sometimes I have up to three seizures in one night, but most often only one. When I become incontinent of urine, my wife usually gets me out of bed and walks me to the bathroom, where she changes my pajamas and dries me off. I am never aware of anything. I wonder where my wife gets the strength to lift me out of bed and take me into the bathroom. I wake up at the usual time in the morning and note that I have on a fresh pair of pajamas and that my old ones and a wet towel are in the bathroom.

75

(*Resident physician*)   I was fresh out of medical school, completing my first year of residency—my internship. If nothing else, at least I had my peace of mind. But which peace did I have? Sleep was something I only dreamt about—daydreamed about, actually. I was dying to have time for myself, although it seemed as though I would die first. I was starving for discipline but satiated with procrastination. I craved french fries and chicken thighs. I fancied fashion but was faithful to my faded green scrubs.

I was weary of looking for someone special to come into my life. The gate was open for my prince and his horse to let themselves in. My lifestyle? Well, I felt lethargic, listless, and lifeless most of the time. The idea of having a family was a completely alien concept. I knew I was aging, which would only buy me automatic membership in Wrinkles Anonymous, Brittle Bones Abound, and finally the Association of the Ascended.

That was my state of mind when, to my surprise, I learned that I had epilepsy.

I had recently become mindful that there were moments when lights would go on in my head, some of them only flickering spikes. But I was just too burned out to think about it. While rotating on the neurology service, I had the opportunity to ask about these quirky episodes of lightheadedness. Who better to ask than a neurologist? I described these 10-second periods during which I experienced a heat rush—a thrill, a charge—throughout my body. "Probably nothing," the neurologist said. After all, I was an otherwise healthy 20-some-thing-year-old brand-spanking-new medical doctor, or so I thought. Wrong!

We continued on rounds, discussing patients (most of whom were admitted for strokes or seizures), and then proceeded to the Radiology Department. It was there that it happened.

I felt that very familiar feeling of apprehension—the premonition. I reached out to the attending neurologist to alert him to what was happening. I felt the shudder and the quiver, without the external trembling, followed by a few moments of apprehension. I held my breath and looked from side to side, as if to get my bearings. "Are you all right?" he asked. I heard him speak but did not attend to it. It was like watching TV while focusing on the heat from a nearby fire. He took my pulse, but it was over. A wave of relaxation swept across me. It was a feeling similar to that of completing a speech in public and then experiencing the loosening of one's muscles from the jaw-clenching tension.

The neurologist pulled me aside from the other members of our ward team and suggested that I have an EEG. What was he thinking? What were the others thinking?

No sooner did I enter the EEG lab than I had an endless number of electrodes applied to my head. Talk about a bad hair day. No wonder the patients returned to the ward looking like the "heat meister." My attending stopped by to see how I was doing, which was comforting. Not so comforting was a visit from the neurology fellow, who was working under the tutelage of the attending. The fellow had stopped by to observe the EEG monitor. What was *he* doing here? I realized that we were in a teaching institution, but I really didn't want to have to face the people with whom I worked. I mean, I didn't know anything about *their* private lives. We had professional, not personal, relationships.

"Well, do you see anything?" I asked. "Yeah, there's something there, but Dr. White (the attending) will talk to you about it." "Something I should be concerned about?" I inquired. "Well, I'll let Dr. White talk to you about it." Oh, that's just great, I thought. What was it? Were the squiggly wigglies wiggling the wrong way? (Note my sophisticated understanding of EEGs.) What could be so bad? I had been having these episodes as far back as I could recall.

At that point I wished I had not brought these spells to anyone's attention. There had been several occasions in the past when the spells occurred while I was in the midst of a group of people and nobody knew, or even during a conversation. Sometimes they occurred so infrequently that I forgot all about them. I think I expected reassurance now that they were nothing to be concerned about, just symptoms of hypoglycemia or stress, perhaps. "We're done," said the technician. "I think Dr. White will see you now."

His first words were, "You have epilepsy."

"Okay. So when will I start flopping around like a fish, doing the piscilian dance?" At least Dr. White reassured me that my seizures could be managed with medication. The mighty medication—"That which will cure you will only make you more tired."

Within a half hour I was sent to have an MRI, a sophisticated procedure that usually takes days to weeks (and relinquishing your firstborn child) to get scheduled. I felt privileged. "Are you the resident who had the seizure during rounds?" asked the MRI tech. Oh, great. Who put out the newsletter, I wondered. Then came 45 minutes of immobilization and listening to the chitty chitty bang bang of the MRI scanning my head. After it was over, I convened with several staff, who took time out of their day to review my brain. No tumor. Heavy sigh. What a relief!

I returned to the neurology ward to see my patients. As I walked down the corridor, groups of physicians and other health-care professionals turned and looked conspicuously at me. "She's the one. There she is." They motioned at me nonchalantly. I met with a fellow resident. "How are you feeling? I heard what happened," he said. I was sorry I missed the broadcast, especially since I was the headliner. Earlier that morning I had been a doctor, a normal person, and now just hours later after being diagnosed with epilepsy I was a patient, feeling like a leper. This was a good test of my character as well as a lesson in medical confidentiality.

As if life wasn't taxing enough, medical school and residency seemed to take away even the simplest of pleasures. Sleep, time, and family had become intangible entities. Dominating my thoughts were feelings of humiliation about my lack of medical knowledge and the fear that I would never acquire it. Now, to add to that, I was told that my brain wasn't working right. Another cross to bear and weight to carry. Somebody give me a crutch.

It has been many months since I have been enlightened about my medical condition. I will be forever grateful to my attending physician and (now) colleague, who has put me at ease, advised me, and reassured me that my children will not necessarily have seizures.

Although this experience has been somewhat unsettling, I have come to realize the following: a seizure is not only a sudden attack of illness. Like it says in the dictionary, to seize is to take possession, to hold firmly, and to arrive at a sudden understanding. I have learned to seize the moment and hold firmly to the understanding that that which does not kill me will make me stronger.

76

(*Nurse*)   A year and a half after undergoing a radical mastectomy, I started experiencing funny spells that were, at the very least, bizarre. I vividly remember my first seizure. It was a warm, sunny day and I was driving through a neighboring village with my three small children in the car. I stopped at a red light, the light changed to green, and I just sat there. A strong, overpowering sense of déjà vu came over me and then a warm, flooding sensation started just below my ribcage, spread into my chest, down my arms, up my neck, and into my head. I felt stunned. Afterwards, I was left with a profound pressure in my head, pressure between my ears, and a sense of confusion.

These episodes were dismissed by my family physician as anxiety. He said, "Just stop taking your thyroid medication." I stopped the medicine but the spells continued. I kept my concern to myself because I didn't want anyone to think I was a neurotic. The spells progressed over the next year, increasing in frequency and intensity. There were different triggers: blinking lights, a passing train, or walking over an iron grate in the sidewalk. Sometimes I couldn't recall what had happened, but the flooding sensation never changed. One day, a year or so later, the spells became very strong and vivid. I felt an overwhelming sense of paranoia and great fear. I recall shopping for groceries and hurrying home because I felt that something bad was going to happen. I wouldn't talk on the phone because I thought that someone was listening in. All the time the spells kept recurring, accompanied by a new component: a smothering, sweet, sticky smell that engulfed my entire head. I lay down on the couch as a wave of exhaustion passed over me. I remember asking my 5-year-old son, "Does Mommy's breath smell funny?" He replied, "No, Mommy, just sleep. I'll take care of you." The last thing I remember that day was reaching for a dish at dinner. Another seizure had occurred.

Some days later, at around 5:00 or 6:00 a.m., my mother was calling me back from a long, dark tunnel. It was difficult to open my eyes, but when I did, I was terrified. There was a man I didn't know drawing up a syringe and another man standing near my husband. "What's wrong? Who are these people? What are they doing?" My husband explained, "It's the doctor and our next door neighbor." My mother said, "You've had another one of your spells, a bad one, but you'll be all right." I had lost all control. I couldn't remember anything—total amnesia. Disoriented and uninhibited, I walked from my bed to the bathroom and sat on the toilet, leaving the door open in front of everyone! I remained very disoriented and extremely tired for the entire day. The only question I remember asking over and over was "What did we have for dinner last night?" I felt that this was the clue to the black hole left in my memory, but the answer didn't help.

My husband never did tell me what happened in bed that morning, but it had a profound effect on him. I returned home from the hospital after 10 days of tests. My husband was told that I had an inoperable tumor and had a year to live—he never told me. My three children were told over and over again, "Don't upset Mommy or she'll get sick." The stress this disorder caused was indescribable. Six years later, my husband and I were divorced. The children have their own memories of scars from that time. I only wish I could take back and absorb the fears I caused them to experience.

It is a terrible feeling to lose a chunk of time in your life and have no control over it. I did not appreciate having that control until I lost it. In retrospect, I feel that this experience changed the way I deal with almost every aspect of my life.

It took many trials of different combinations of anticonvulsants before my seizures became controlled. Those years were some of the most terrifying times of my life. Each time a seizure broke through, I was fearful that I would have another grand mal. I did not want to leave the house. When I explained my fears to my physician, he said, "Oh, just sit down on the curb so you won't get hurt" and then laughed. His dismissal of my fears has remained with me, but the hurt and anger subsided after I switched to another doctor. Today my seizures are well controlled, although I still have occasional déjà vu episodes. There are occasional brief lapses of time that I notice afterwards, but they don't interfere with my life.

I returned to school and obtained a degree in nursing. After 12 years in a clinical setting, I joined a neurologic practice and embarked on one of the most challenging and exciting ventures of my life, one that involved coordinating trials of new epilepsy drugs.

Once, while I was conducting a battery of neuropsychological tests, the patient paused, took a breath, and explained that she had just experienced a seizure. She quietly said, "You'll think I am crazy," and proceeded to describe her seizure. As she spoke I could hardly believe my ears: her seizure mirrored mine. I told her that I, too, had epilepsy and that my seizures were very similar to hers. In that moment we had validated many of the unspoken feelings and fears of persons who have epilepsy. Is this real? Could it be something else? Do other people have these same feelings? Why me? We cried a few tears and laughed a lot more over the bizarre paths our lives had taken. This experience brought to mind the time immediately after my mastectomy when, at the age of 29, I asked the nurse, "What will I do? What will I wear?" She replied, "Well, honey, here's what I do," and she pulled a prosthesis out of her bra! I couldn't believe it. She didn't look any different from any other woman. The nurse gave me back my sense of being whole. I realized that I was no different from anyone else. From that day forward I have treasured those moments of sharing. I had simply experienced a different turn in my life.

It was this same sense of reaching out and sharing that I felt with this woman with epilepsy. Putting these experiences into perspective has made me realize how important it is to share my experiences with others so that they do not have to feel alone, frightened, or misunderstood.

These experiences have carried me throughout my life and allowed me to reach out in a unique way to some of our patients and families who have been most devastated by epilepsy. In some ways, I regard my seizure disorder as just another tool I've been given with which to reach out and help others.

77

(*Neurologist*) My journey with epilepsy has been easier than those taken by many of my patients. I was 9 years old and singing along with the rest of the congregation in church one Sunday when my vision suddenly went black and I lost consciousness. I awoke in the minister's study. How did I get there? Piles of paper were scattered across his large desk and spilled onto the floor. Row upon row of dusty old books were neatly placed, the shelves rising to the ceiling.

My mother was holding me. I could tell she had been crying. Her eyelids were puffy and her eyes streaked with red. Her makeup was smeared. A woman who sat behind us in church was wiping my face with a towel.

I felt dazed and drained, and unable to concentrate. The time on the clock was 30 minutes later than it should have been. My mother was quiet. The other woman explained, "It is going to be okay. I am a nurse and I helped bring you in here. You had a seizure." My thoughts were confused. Who are you? Why isn't my mother talking? She looks so scared. Did *I* scare my mother?

Mom then explained that I had stiffened out, drooled, and shaken all over for a minute. Dad came in and picked me up. He kissed me and smiled, and I fell asleep. I do not remember the rest of that day. I woke up at home in my bed.

Later that week my mother and I went to see a neurologist. His waiting room was large. I liked all the magazines scattered on tables, and Mom tried to keep me still. It was more fun looking at the pictures than thinking about what was to come. When I was called back to the doctor's office, I became frightened. What was a neurologist? What was he going to do? The office itself was small. The doctor had thin, gray hair and wore eyeglasses. He sat behind a large oak desk. The desk was so huge I could barely look over the edge to see his face. There was a window, and I remember passing the time looking outside, trying to find our car in the parking lot while my mother talked. "No, he has never done this in the past. No, no one in the family has epilepsy. No, he never had seizures with fever when he was a baby. Well, he did fall down the basement steps when he was 2 years old and was knocked out briefly, but he has never had a seizure before."

The doctor appeared very large to me and held my hand as he walked me to an exam room. He checked my reflexes, which I thought was pretty neat. He had me walk heel to toe and tested my strength and balance. He walked me back to my mother and said he wanted us to come back later in the week for an EEG and then to see him again.

Later that week I went for my first EEG. The technician put needle electrodes all over my scalp. I winced several times. Luckily, needle electrodes are seldom used today. I hated the deep breathing part because it made me feel cold and tingly. When it was over, the technician told me not to comb my hair because my scalp might start bleeding. I went back to the waiting room and sat by my mother. A few minutes later I felt a warm trickle on my neck. My mother ran and got a towel. I had scratched my scalp, and a small amount of blood had run onto my shirt collar. It quickly stopped and we went in to see the doctor.

The technician laid the EEG on his desk. He stood up and flipped through the paper. Every few pages he paused but did not say anything. I got up and peered over the top of the desk to look at the paper. "There is a spike," he said and showed me a pointy squiggle. That sounded bad to me; I did not know what a spike was or meant. He finished looking at the EEG and gave my mother a prescription for seizure medication for me to take.

The only problem was that the medication caused me to have swollen gums, no matter how much I brushed and flossed. But it was manageable. I wondered if the seizure was going to happen again. I wondered if people had seizures and died. What would my mother and father do if I died? I had thoughts that a 9-year-old should not have. I took the medication every night and did okay until a year later.

It was a hot day in the first week of July, and I was mowing the backyard. Our backyard had a slope that went down past some apple trees to a drainage ditch. I always started up next to the house and mowed back and forth toward the bottom of the hill. Two-thirds of the way down the hill I suddenly passed out. It was the same blackness that had overcome me in church. I lost control of my arms and legs, and went down. I awoke lying on the ground and saw that I had landed in the shade of an apple tree. I heard the lawnmower roaring a few feet from where I lay. Who was controlling the lawnmower? I turned over and realized that no one was. It was stuck against the fence at the bottom of the hill but was still running. In those days there was no safety handle that automatically turned off the lawnmower when released.

Then there was a noise from the house. Crash! The back screen door slammed shut. My mother ran across the yard yelling for someone to turn off the lawnmower. No one was there except me. I tried to get up but felt too tired. Mother looked scared to death and quickly made sure the lawnmower had not cut off my hand or foot, which it had not. It was all I could do to get into the house. I felt exhausted, as if I had run a marathon. The couch felt good and I fell asleep. I still do not know who turned off the lawnmower.

A few days later, on the Fourth of July during a volleyball game, it happened once again. Our team was ahead. Smack! I hit the ball over the net. Then nothing. I awoke to a crowd of sweaty bodies standing over me. The sun was blinding, and I could not make out any of the faces. Family members frantically parted the onlookers and took me to lie down in a nylon webbed lounge chair. Occasionally someone came by to see if I was okay. Others glanced at me in fear and would not come close. Surrounded by people, I felt alone. My parents took me home. I did not understand why people were afraid of seeing someone have a seizure. And I did not understand why I had two seizures that week. I was taking my medicine correctly. What was wrong?

We went back to the neurologist. He had me undergo another EEG. This time I kept my hand away from my hair and got no blood on my collar. I stood in front of his desk and looked across it as he flipped through my EEG. "Are there any spikes?" I asked. "Yes, quite a few," he replied. I had gained a few pounds in the past year, and my seizure drug level was low. My dose was adjusted upward. I brushed my teeth more often.

I never had another seizure. My dose of seizure medication remained the same for 4 years. At 14 years of age I weighed more than I had at 10, and I am sure my serum level was again low. But rather than increase the dose, my neurologist tapered me off the medication over the next several months. One year later he told me that he did not have to see me anymore. Mom seemed happy.

Several years later, I entered medical school and then did a neurology residency. Now I am finishing an epilepsy fellowship.

Because of my own experiences, I have, perhaps, an uncommon perspective on epilepsy. Epilepsy has not yet left my personal life. My EEG continues to show generalized spike discharges. I know this can be an inherited trait. I look at my healthy 6-month-old son and wonder.

I see a lot of EEGs and patients with epilepsy. Parents often arrive in the office with faces full of fear and apprehension, clutching their children as if holding on for dear life. At those times, I often think of my mother and the look on her face the day I had a seizure in church and the day she feared the lawnmower had cut off my foot.

And I understand.

Appendix

Story Authors

❖ ❖ ❖ ❖ ❖

Mary Alice Bare, R.N., M.S.P.H.

Gregory L. Barkley, M.D.

Elinor Ben-Menachem, M.D., Ph.D.

Joseph Bruni, M.D.

David Burdette, M.D.

Joan Callery, R.N.

Julie Carpenter, R.N.

Enrique J. Carrazana, M.D.

David Chadwick, D.M., F.R.C.P.

Harvey S. Cooper, R.N.

Joyce Cramer

Mogens Dam, M.D.

Cecile Davis

Orrin Devinsky, M.D.

Alan B. Ettinger, M.D.

Robert S. Fisher, M.D., Ph.D.

Gail Fromes, R.N., M.S.

Barbara Rader Gahry, C.M.A., M.S.W.

Janet Gentile, R.N.

James Grisolia, M.D.

Cynthia Harden, M.D.

Susan L. Harper

Edward J. Hart, M.D.

Jeanette C. Hartshorn, R.N., Ph.D., F.A.A.N.

Diane Healy, R.N.

Peggy Hugger, R.N.

John R. Hughes, M.D., Ph.D.

Peter W. Kaplan, M.B., F.R.C.P.

Lissa Robins Kapust, L.I.C.S.W.

Sookyong Koh, M.D., Ph.D.

K. Babu Krishnamurthy, M.D.

David M. Labiner, M.D.

Marcelo Lancman, M.D.

Cynthia Lehan, O.T.

Brian Litt, M.D.

David Longmire, M.D.

Harry Meinardi, M.D., Ph.D

Beth Malow, M.D.

Christine Moan, R.N.

Georgia D. Montouris, M.D.

John M. Pellock, M.D.

Patricia E. Penovich, M.D.

Michael Privitera, M.D.

Guy Remillard, M.D.

Janet Rowe, R.N.

Eileen Salmonson, L.I.C.S.W.

Joseph I. Sirven, M.D.

Dieter Schmidt, M.D.

Brien J. Smith, M.D.

Cathy Smith, R.N.

Elizabeth B. Sullivan, M.S.

Tracey Thomas

Paolo Tinuper, M.D.

David Vossler, M.D.

Anita K. Wagner, Pharm.D.

Braxton B. Wannamaker, M.D.

Andrew N. Wilner, M.D.

Robert G. Ziegler, M.D.